Taking Care of Precious Ones

taking care of precious ones

carrie neckien
m.a., ccls

Cover layout and book design by
Christopher Green Design
christophergreen.com

Printed in the United States of America

10 9 8 7 6 5 4 3 2 1

This book is dedicated to the children I have met in my lifetime who have shown me how precious the life of a child truly is.

And to my family and friends who have offered their undying support of me and my life's work.

Mark

Mark and his family had traveled to Korea for the wedding of a family friend, with plans to have the vacation of a lifetime. They had so many things they wanted to do and so many sights to see. One morning on their trip, they set out to go to Myung-Dong district when suddenly a car jumped the curb and was heading right for them. Mark reacted without hesitation and pushed his family out of the way. He was hit by the car and was left unresponsive on the side of the curb. Katie, Mark's wife, turned around and saw Mark lying there unconscious. Shortly thereafter, an ambulance arrived on the scene and took Mark, who was still unconscious, to a nearby hospital. Katie and the kids were unable to ride with him.

VIII | taking care of precious ones

Mark was immediately triaged in the ambulance. After a short time, his eyes opened in terror. He had no idea where he was and was startled by the strangers who hovered over him. He looked frantically for his family members, who were nowhere to be seen. Adding to Mark's confusion and panic was the immense pain he felt in his legs. He was barely conscious and was utterly confused. He began fighting off the ambulance workers because he thought that they were trying to hurt him. The next thing he knew, his arms and legs were being restrained. He screamed and fought helplessly against the two ambulance workers who were holding him down.

Mark continued to be extremely agitated and frantically kept asking where his wife and children were. After receiving some sort of injection, however, Mark started to calm. It was then that he realized he was in an ambulance. He began trying to formulate his thoughts to ask questions about what had happened to him and where his family was. He was exasperated and felt hopeless, as he was unable to communicate with the ambulance workers. They were speaking Korean and did not seem to know any English at all. It sounded like they were asking him some questions, but he couldn't be sure. He could not understand them, and his frustration was heightened by the immense amount of pain he felt and the fear that overwhelmed him as he thought of his family. *Where they hurt too? Were they even alive?*

The ambulance worker kept repeating himself, attempting to communicate and help Mark understand what was going on. Mark was still disoriented but was slowly beginning to remember what had happened. He envisioned an out-of-control car and his family screaming, but that was all he could recall. In this aggravated state of mind, he remained uncooperative. He kept resisting the help the ambulance worker was offering him, trying to swat away the needle and syringe that were in the worker's hand. It felt as if he were handcuffed to the sides of the bed. As he screamed and pleaded to be let up, his efforts were ignored, and the ambulance proceeded to what looked like a hospital, yet its name and location were unknown to him. Mark was terrified that he would never see his family again.

At the hospital, Mark remained terrified as he was being examined. His clothes were taken off, he was being poked and prodded by medical instruments that he had never seen before, and people in uniforms (which he assumed were doctors and nurses) were moving quickly around him. Each person was speaking in a foreign language and touching him with one thing or another. Mark was begging for answers and praying for someone who spoke English. Nobody seemed to hear his request. It was lucky for them that he was still restrained!

Finally, after what seemed like hours, Katie and the kids arrived at Mark's bedside. Tears overcame him; he was so thankful and relieved. Now that Mark knew his family was safe and they were together again, the situation seemed much more tolerable to him.

He became more cooperative and allowed the doctors to do what they needed to. Katie was able to tell him what happened, and this knowledge was helpful to Mark. It helped him make sense of what the doctors were doing to him, explained some of the need for all the tests and the IV tubes, and gave reason for the pain he was feeling. He still felt nervousness and a discomfort that he had never felt before. He was completely at the mercy of these people who were not able to explain what they were doing to him. The uncertainty and unpredictability were unbearable, and all Mark wanted to do was go home with his family. He wished he had never come to Korea and vowed to never leave home again. Although this may not seem like a rational reaction, we can all relate to the fears this experience aroused in Mark.

This story of Mark and his family communicates a valuable lesson and gives us a vivid picture of how children feel in the medical environment. Just imagine how it would feel to be hurt and scared, with no one to talk to or ask questions. Although little patients may speak the language and have their parents present, children are usually excluded from the conversations held about their medical condition. Doctors and nurses typically address the parents, speaking to the child much less frequently.

When they do speak to the child, they often use words that children do not understand and unintentionally use words that are threatening to them (we will discuss this in Chapter 6).

The fact is that the medical environment is like a foreign place to children, whether they speak the language or not. They feel *exactly* like Mark did when he was injured in Korea. They do not understand the terminology the staff uses, like a foreign language. Having never seen medical instruments before, children do not know what they are or what they are used for, and they wonder which of these instruments are going to hurt them. As a result, children show fear of almost everything they have never seen before. They are afraid of tongue depressors, ear curettes, nasal suction bulbs, even tape. This list goes on and on! More times than not, children who have not had any experience in the medical environment or have not had the benefit of age-appropriate education and preparation begin to cry and seem irrational to their parents. Parents try to control their children's reactions so their children do not embarrass them.

Often parents use empty threats or belittle a child's fears when the child is "acting out" at the doctor's.

When parents do this, children view them as being on the doctor's side, playing against them on Team "Grown up" or Team "You better behave yourself or else." Children feel alone and like they are being overpowered. Their growing independence and their esteem are shattered as they feel their voice isn't heard and their opinion does not matter. Their fears and feelings of helplessness consume them. At this point, they are unable to listen to reason, their behaviors are difficult to redirect, and it becomes nearly impossible for them to trust someone enough to help them cope effectively. Ultimately, all they feel is fear and helplessness. This is what leaves children traumatized by the medical environment!

The purpose of this book is to help parents understand how to help their children through threatening situations, particularly at the doctor's office, emergency room, or hospital. My suggestions not only will help in the medical arena, but also will teach parents how to help their children cope with any stressful or anxiety-evoking situation that could occur in their everyday lives. I hope to help raise a generation of adults who are unafraid of the medical environment, free of those horrific stories many have to tell about their first experiences with pain and doctors.

contents

Zachery and Justin

What is the first memory you have of the doctor or the hospital? Is it a pleasant one? I would guess that your answer is likely, "No." Most of us have a story to tell about a medical experience we had when we were kids. My story is vivid. I remember every detail, and I don't think I will ever forget.

My first memory of pain happened when I was four years old. My brother and I were outside playing and we found a cereal bowl, which of course I proceeded to throw at him. In retaliation, he pushed me and I fell onto a split brick and sliced open my arm. My mom rushed me to the doctor. However, when we arrived I didn't know the doctor on duty (my regular doctor was not there), and I didn't know how bad my injury was. I was scared. I saw the doctor fill a syringe, and as he turned toward me with it, I lost it. I kicked, screamed, and wrestled with the nurse until she had to call another nurse for help. In total, it took four nurses to restrain me, and the only thing that made me calm down was when they threatened to make my mom leave the room if I didn't stop. The nurses held me down as the doctor gave me a shot and stitched up my arm. I received 23 stitches that day. Their tactic worked as it forced me to calm down, but it left a traumatized little girl who grew up afraid of the doctor, afraid of shots, and uneasy in new situations.

I believe that if someone had taken the time to explain what was happening and had told me step-by-step what the doctor was going to do, if they had supported me or distracted me during the visit instead of holding me down against my will, I'll bet my memory of that event would be much more positive. Today at 33 years of age, I would not have a stinging memory of that day when I was four.

For 10 years, I have worked in an inpatient pediatric setting as a certified Child Life Specialist. My job is to help children cope with the medical environment. I prepare and teach children in a way that is appropriate for their age and stage of development. This involves helping them cope with the experience so they leave the medical center without stress or trauma caused by fear, pain, or misconception about medical events. Ultimately, I have the task of supporting children and families throughout their medical experience and making it as easy for them as possible.

The medical setting is unwelcoming to children. The décor caters to adults who expect a sterile hospital environment, and there is typically only a very small place for the children to play, if there is any place at all. Children are fearful of the hospital for many reasons. Many associate the hospital with pain and needles or even death and dying. Because the hospital milieu is totally unfamiliar to them, children experience a high level of anxiety as a result of fears of the unknown, stranger anxiety, separation anxiety, and lack of independence and procedural knowledge.

In my job, I have seen the effect of negative hospital experiences on countless children. The fear that can manifest as a result of a child's first experience with the doctor and the hospital can have lasting effects on his view of the medical profession. Many of these negative reactions could be avoided if children's fears and experiences were addressed appropriately. In my years of on-the-job experience, I have provided valuable support to children through play, preparation, distraction, and teaching of coping techniques.

Unfortunately, there is not a Child Life Specialist in every hospital and medical environment. In fact, the vast majority of our population doesn't even know what a Child Life Specialist is or understand the value in the profession. My goal with this book is to help you and your family—and by extension, many families— because the more people like you who know about the profession, the more you will ask your doctors for this kind of support. When the need is identified, hospital administrations will be more willing to fund positions for Child Life Specialists. My desire is to have at least one Child Life Specialist position created in every pediatric setting to support children and families during difficult medical situations.

Zachery

Zachery is my son. He is a four-year-old boy who has had many interactions with doctors and medical professionals. Some of these experiences have been more difficult than others in that some of them resulted in him experiencing pain. He has had tubes placed in his ears twice. He has been scoped through the nose. He has had a tonsillectomy and an adenoidectomy, multiple ER visits, an anaphylactic reaction to a peanut allergy, asthma, allergies, eczema, many ear infections, injections, multiple lab draws, and immunizations. Regardless of all these and the pain he has experienced, he loves his doctor. How is this possible?

I have found that the key to this trusting relationship with his doctor is the result of a few things. First and foremost, Zachery age-appropriately understands the doctor's role in his life. He comprehends that whenever parts of his body are not working correctly, he goes to see his doctor, who will help fix him and give him the right medicine to make him feel better. He trusts that although doctors sometimes have to perform procedures or tests that are uncomfortable, foreign to him, or painful, his doctor is looking out for him and wants him to feel better. He feels the same way toward his mom.

Second, Zachery also relies on the knowledge that his mom will help him through the experience. He has been taught to cope with fear and pain. He trusts that his mom is going to tell him the truth about what he will experience, even if it will hurt or be uncomfortable. Zachery knows wholeheartedly that his mom will be there to support him throughout whatever he is going through; she will acknowledge and understand his feelings, provide emotional support, give hugs and kisses, and offer reassurance. My hope is that this book will help you develop this kind of trusting relationship with your child. This type of relationship with you will enable your child to have better experiences in the medical environment, including at the doctor's office, dentist's office, and hospital. I want medical experiences to be minimally stressful for children and families. Your relationship with your child should never need to be compromised as the result of a doctor's visit or a trip to the dentist during which your child experiences such fear and anxiety that he leaves feeling traumatized.

Throughout my career, I have worked with many fearful children and terrified parents. I have seen a broad spectrum of reactions to the medical environment, ranging from smiles to screams. One of the first children with whom I ever worked, at the beginning of my career, was on the opposite end of this spectrum from Zachery. I will call him Justin.

Justin

Justin was a five-year-old boy with a comprehensive medical history. He had been hospitalized multiple times and had many procedures that had traumatized him. As a result, Justin screamed and cried whenever he had to go to the doctor's office. He was uncooperative with his parents and the doctor and was resistant and combative throughout the duration of his visits. He had to be held down for simple procedures like the measuring of his blood pressure and taking of his temperature. He required sedation for minimally invasive procedures; this takes much more time and often delays the procedure because sedation requires a Pediatric Intensive Care Unit (PICU) bed or an outpatient surgical team. For Justin and his parents, the medical environment had become a place of anxiety and fear. Justin typically left feeling panicked, distrustful, and emotionally and physically exhausted. These experiences were just as difficult for his parents.

It is my belief that every mom and dad wants the best for their children and would love some tools to help their child when he is suffering or scared. The majority of the parents with whom I have worked are overwhelmingly accepting of information that will make medical experiences and hospitalization easier for their children. Let's take Justin's mom, for example. She doesn't know how to help her son cope with his medical experiences or how to make him behave when he visits the doctor. She is embarrassed both by his behavior and by her inability to control him during the doctor visits. This embarrassment typically leads to anger, and she gets mad at Justin for not listening to her or cooperating. She tried parenting him the best she knew how. She focused on trying to control immediate behaviors (such as crying, hitting, and kicking) and to stop his tantrums. In fact, when I first met her, I learned that she had tricked Justin to get him to the hospital. To her this seemed like the perfect thing to say to him, "Let's go to the toy store." Justin got in the car without protest and didn't cry on the way to the doctor's office. This scenario played out well for Justin's mom, until he arrived at the hospital and realized where he was.

You can imagine Justin's reaction. He screamed, cried, and had to be carried into the office against his will. He hit his mother and yelled and screamed at her. His behavior was irrational to the onlooker, but behind this tantrum is truly an age-appropriate reaction to fear, distrust, and disappointment. Justin was devastated, and he had a right to be. What child wouldn't be? Imagine for a moment, walking in Justin's shoes, thinking that you are about to go to a toy store to get a new toy, only to be blindsided and dragged into a doctor's office, where you didn't know why you were there or what they were going to do to you. Not only that, but consider being lied to by the one person you want to trust the most. The first thing you would think is, *"Why am I here? Are they going to hurt me? Why do I have to come here? What did I do wrong to make my parent take me here?"* That feeling of being misled or lied to is a hurtful and scary feeling for all of us, no matter how old we are.

Once parents realize that their words and level of support can affect the outcome of their child's medical experiences, they most often want to learn how to attain the knowledge to do so. Stories like Justin's make it easier to understand and sympathize with our children and aspire to learn how to give our children the tools necessary to cope effectively with medical visits and procedures. Once children lose trust in their primary caregiver, it makes it extremely difficult to help them trust their environment and cope effectively with anxiety-inducing situations. This can potentially affect them for the rest of their lives.

Medical experiences can be made easier for a child. I believe that children need the following EIGHT things to facilitate a positive experience in the medical setting. These basic principles—explained in the chapters of this book—will help you, as a parent, understand what your child needs to cope effectively and to avoid negative, traumatic experiences.

What Do Children Need?

1. *Age-appropriate introductions to the doctor and medical environment. A chapter on relationship building (**Frank**).*

2. *Tools to cope with heightened anxiety and fear. A chapter on trust (**Brayden**).*

3. *A strong tower of trust, or a trusting relationship with a parent/caregiver. A chapter on tools for coping (**Jaime**).*

4. *The feeling that their voice is being heard and understood. A chapter on listening and providing empathy (**Gregory**).*

5. *Developmentally appropriate education and communication about medical events. A chapter on introducing medical procedures (**Jonathan**).*

6. *Step-by-step preparation about their experiences. A chapter on providing the detailed information to children of all ages in a non-threatening way (**Amy**).*

7. *The opportunity to play. A chapter on play and its necessity (**Carrie**).*

8. *The use of positive reinforcement and rewards. A chapter on rewarding desired behaviors* **(Zachery)**.

Chapter 1

An Age-Appropriate Introduction to the Doctor and Medical Environments

Frank

From infancy, children visit the doctor on a regular basis. As they grow and develop, they begin to remember previous visits and are able to recall painful experiences. Children can begin to associate negative experiences with the medical environment if they are not appropriately prepared for their visits. Children of all ages require an age-appropriate introduction to their doctor and the medical environment. From infancy, children need positive reinforcement surrounding the medical environment. This must be an ongoing process; as the child grows, it will get more complex, like being given pieces to a puzzle slowly, as they are able to comprehend more, until one day they are capable of seeing the big picture. Children need constant reminders that doctors are their friends. They need a positive perception and understanding of a doctor's job. Young children are capable of comprehending that a doctor's job is to keep them healthy and to help when their bodies are not working right. A pediatrician's intent is to help children grow and develop into healthy, happy adults, and it is a parent's job to help children understand that concept.

How do you get your child to that level of understanding? Here are a few tips to help facilitate an age-appropriate introduction:

1. Introduce the topic in a safe environment, like during play.

2. Guide play experiences.

3. Introduce, teach, and practice coping skills.

First, to introduce the medical environment to your child, approach the subject in a safe place, like during play. Not only do children learn and listen best during play, the play environment is a safe place for them because it is where they have the tools they need to cope effectively. You can buy a medical kit and a pretend doctor's uniform at the local toy store. Spend quiet time playing with your child in this activity. This is the perfect opportunity to engage your child in playful learning, without the need for direct dialogue about the doctor or the visit. You can easily introduce medical instruments by playing with them. The toys provide you with the tools necessary to help you discuss what your child will experience during a doctor's visit. Show her what the play tools are, verbally label them for the child, and demonstrate what each item and instrument does and what its purposes are. Then, while at the doctor's visit, you can remind your child about the play experiences. For example, "Look, the doctor is going to use a stethoscope; you have a red one at home. Remember when you listened to Mommy's heartbeat to hear if it was working right? The doctor is going to listen to your heartbeat now." Follow up by saying, "How does _____'s heart sound, Doctor?"

Furthermore, these types of guided play experiences and medical play toys will allow for role play, which is so vital to a child's understanding of the doctor's involvement in his life. Allow your child to play the role of the doctor and/or the patient. In doing so, you will be able to learn about what your child knows and thinks about the doctor. Use this valuable information to talk to your child, correct misconceptions, and teach him how to cope with things that he identifies as scary. Role play can also show you what your little one thinks of the doctor and medical procedures. I have played with some children who are fixated on the play syringe. They love giving shots and typically will give shots repeatedly and as a punishment. They stab the play syringe into their pretend patient and use it as a way to hurt their patient, often saying things like, "You were bad." Comments like these can identify that your child recalls a painful experience with a needle and possibly feels that the shot was given as a punishment. Children who have memories like this need some age-appropriate education about shots and their purpose, and they need to be taught how to cope with getting an injection. This process can be challenging because the child already had a negative experience, but his thoughts and feelings about the process can improve. Children can definitely learn to better cope with painful experiences.

Early in my career working as a Child Life Specialist, a child was admitted to our hospital who was a victim of the devastating earthquake in Turkey in 2003. This earthquake rocked Turkey and killed many people there. Frank was a patient of mine. His pregnant mother was killed in the tragedy trying to protect him. Frank and his family were buried in rubble and were unable to move. When they were rescued a few days later, his mother was found hovered over the top of him, dead. His legs were injured badly and needed surgery and skin grafting. The flesh was torn from his leg so far down that his bone was visible. Frank and his father were brought to this country for treatment by a loving aunt and uncle. Frank was four and didn't speak any English.

I vividly remember feeling that I was not capable of helping this boy. I worried about the language barrier and believed that he needed much more support than I could offer. I felt as if I were in over my head and did not know how to approach the issue of his mother's death to support him through the process of grieving her. This boy taught me something very profound: Play is a universal language. We didn't need words.

I visited Frank daily, and each time, I brought him another toy or project. At our first meeting, I provided many toys because he had nothing but clothing with him. This made me a friend to him immediately. We played and created with playdough, a sensory activity that he loved. Frank was smiling and getting the opportunity to play and act like a kid while in pain and during a time of suffering. He frequented the playroom when he was stable enough to use a wheelchair. During one play session, we were playing with a beach ball, bumping it back and forth to each other. When we finished this activity, I was looking in the cabinets for the next game we'd try. When I turned around, Frank had the ball under his shirt, rubbing it as if it were a baby. I was nearly in tears, yet I reached for a bucket of crayons and paper. I began drawing a picture of a house. He quickly followed suit and began drawing his house and pictures of his family.

He cried, and I did too. His father put the picture up in his room, and as he learned more and more English, he was able to tell me the story behind Frank's picture. I am sure that to this day, that picture drawn by his four-year-old is a treasure to his father.

For children, this kind of catharsis can be reached most easily in play. It was Frank's avenue for communication. Through pictures, role play, pretend, and modeling, we were able to show Frank that we cared about him and wanted to help him when he felt scared or sad. He liked to spend time in the playroom, away from his patient room and away from the nurses and doctors. That playroom was his safe place, the only place where he could do what he knew, to just play.

Just Playing
by Anita Wadley
(*Chicken Soup for the Unsinkable Soul – reprinted with permission*)

When I'm building in the block room,
Please don't say I'm "Just playing."

For, you see, I'm learning as I play,
About balance, I may be an architect someday.

When I'm getting all dressed up,
Setting the table, caring for the babies,
Don't get the idea I'm "Just Playing."
I may be a mother or a father someday.

When you see me up to my elbows in paint,
Or standing at an easel, or molding and shaping clay,
Please don't let me hear you say, "He is Just Playing."
For, you see, I'm learning as I play.
I just might be a teacher someday.

When you see me engrossed in a puzzle
Or some "playing" at my school,
Please don't feel the time is wasted in "play."
For you see, I'm learning as I play.
I'm learning to solve problems and concentrate.
I may be in business someday.

When you see me cooking or tasting foods,
Please don't think that because I enjoy it, it is "Just Play."
I'm learning to follow directions and see the differences.
I may be a cook someday.

When you see me learning to skip, hop, run, and move my

body,
Please don't say I'm "Just Playing."
For, you see, I'm learning as I play.
I'm learning how my body works.
I may be a doctor, nurse, or athlete someday.

When you ask me what I've done at school today,
And I say, "I just played."
Please don't misunderstand me.
For, you see, I'm learning as I play.
I'm learning to enjoy and be successful in my work.
I'm preparing for tomorrow.
Today, I am a child and my work is play.

Finally, some effective coping skills to introduce are deep breathing exercises, distraction, guided imagery, and relaxation exercises. All of these will be discussed in greater detail in the next chapter. Once you teach these skills, practice them so that your child will be able to utilize these new skills during times of heightened anxiety, at the doctor's office, before a shot, or before any kind of procedure. If you rehearse various coping skills with your child, you will be able to determine the methods she is most comfortable with. Once your child finds a coping skill that works best for him, always be prepared to provide him with the tools he needs to cope successfully. For example, if your child likes to distract himself during stressful times, then make sure you bring a "distracter" to the doctor's office for him. This "distracter" could be a book, a small video game system (like a DS or a PSP), a View Finder, a coloring page, and so on. If your child chooses to get involved in guided imagery (explained in Chapter 2), make sure that the person taking your child to his doctor's visit is able to lead him or guide him through the imagery. If the child likes to participate in deep breathing exercises, bubbles or pinwheels are great to facilitate the breathing exercise. Imagining he is blowing out birthday candles is a great tool as well. This works well for the school-age child. The point is, the parent or caregiver needs to take the responsibility off the child's fearful little shoulders and take this job on himself or herself. Let the child know you are there for him to help him through stressful times. These coping skills can be implemented and are an excellent tool to use throughout all ages and stages of your child's life, not just in medical situations.

Going beyond an introduction to the medical environment, giving your child age-appropriate education is also important. Talking about age-appropriate education can be confusing. The way you talk to a seven-year-old sounds completely different from the way you talk to a three-year-old. The problem is, how do you know how much information is enough, without giving too much or too little? If you give too much information, a child may become unnecessarily afraid; if you don't give enough, it could make her feel like you are not telling the truth or are keeping a secret. I have found this to be a good rule of thumb: Speak in sentences that are the same number of words as the child is old, plus two. For example, a two-year-old could be spoken to in four-word sentences. If it's much more than that, there is a good chance that the child will not comprehend the entirety of what you are trying to convey to her. So, first, speak in sentences that are the same number of words as the child is old, plus two.

Second, allow the child to guide you. Start simply; ask questions that allow the child to tell you what he knows. For example, "You are going to have surgery tomorrow. Do you know what surgery is?" and "What do you think that means?" Build your explanations slowly. Sometimes this means stopping and revisiting the topic another time, another day even. If a child understands you, you will know. He will be able to answer questions to confirm his understanding. You could ask, "So, are you going to be asleep or awake for your surgery?" and "Is it going to hurt?" Then reaffirm and reassure the child, "No, it is not going to hurt because you are going to be asleep the whole time," adding later, "It may hurt when you wake up, but Mommy will be there to kiss it and help you however you need to make it better."

Last, make sure you give your child an open door for communication, so he feels that he is able to ask anything! Allow for questions, and before you answer, make sure you know the answer. If you don't, be honest with the child, and tell him you don't know. Tell your child that you don't know the answer to the question, but you will be able to get an answer from the doctor when you get to the hospital. Make sure you remember to ask the doctor those questions to show your child that his concerns are valid and important. By doing this, you are communicating that you are on his side, and you are trying to alleviate his fears.

A good way to do this is to give the child a little communication notebook to write down his questions, which you will take to the doctor's office or hospital. This is a good way to show your child that you care and are trying to meet his needs (and it will help you not forget the questions). It is a great tool for parents as well. We so easily get caught up in an appointment or admission. We are so overwhelmed by the experience that when the doctor walks in, we listen to what he or she has to say, while at the same time, we try to provide comfort and age-appropriate information to our children. It leaves little time for us to think about what questions we wanted to ask. I cannot count the times I left the doctor's office frustrated that I forgot to ask the question I intended to ask. Often it is not easy to get in touch with a doctor once you have left the office. For this reason, a communication book is a great idea, for both children and parents.

Chapter 1 Review

1. *Children can begin to associate negative experiences with the medical environment if they are not appropriately prepared for their visits.*

2. *Children of all ages require an age-appropriate introduction to their doctor and the medical environment through play and age- appropriate education.*

3. *Speak in sentences that are the same number of words as the child is old, plus two.*

Tools to Cope with Heightened Anxiety and Fear

Brayden

There are different ways to help children through situations of heightened anxiety and fear. I have found the most effective coping skills for children are distraction, deep breathing, guided imagery, and sensory stimulation. Every child will prefer something different, and because of those preferences, you need to identify the child's style of coping prior to the medical visit.

It is important to keep in mind that all children cope differently. Some children seek information. Others avoid it. You can determine the type of coping your child prefers simply by talking to her about an upcoming event. Does your child want all the juicy details and to talk about situations in depth? Or is your child difficult to engage in conversation, giving you one-word answers and appearing to ignore you when you are talking about serious situations?

"**Information seekers**" ask a lot of questions and typically want to watch everything. These children like to see preparation materials, reading them thoroughly. They engage in deep conversation and question every procedure and its purpose. These are the kids who walk around with an anatomy doll or book. They observe the nurse inquisitively and must watch as she performs her duties, whether changing a dressing or starting an IV.

"**Avoiders**" do not want to engage in conversation about their medical situation or procedures. They change the subject when confronted with information they do not want to hear. These children also typically do not want to watch a procedure being done and tend to withdraw when a nurse or doctor enters the room. They will typically not make eye contact with the person who is perceived to be threatening and will close their eyes or look away when a threatening instrument or medical device is presented.

I personally am an avoider; watching or listening to someone who is preparing me for something medical just makes me more anxious. I dwell on the thought of pain and concentrate on just how miserable the pain is or will be. To explain just how much of an avoider I am, I will share another little story with you. I had to have surgery when I was about 20 years old. I didn't want to know about any of the preparation for the surgery. I asked the doctor to explain it to my dad instead. If I had listened, I know that I would have imagined the surgery, the slicing and dicing, and that would have done me more harm than good. I knew that I would be better off showing up to the surgery, getting my IV, and just going to sleep. I was scared then and remained afraid of the medical environment until I became a Child Life Specialist. I watched many brave children undergo much more intensive treatments and painful procedures than I had ever imagined. A light just clicked on in my head; I realized, *If these little kids can do this, so can I.* I went through a period of embarrassment and realized that I had nothing to fear and certainly nothing to complain about.

Once you have figured out whether your child is an avoider or an information seeker, you can then help him identify which of the four major coping techniques would be best suited for him during times of being scared or stressed. Typically, distraction and sensory stimulation work well with avoiders and children who have trouble focusing. Deep breathing and guided imagery work well for children who are more mature and introspective; information seekers typically fit this description. That being said, the majority of the pediatric populations with whom I have worked, who are scared and unsure of their surroundings, are avoiders.

In this chapter, you will read about each coping skill in detail, and I will give you tips on how to use them. Once you identify your child's preferred coping style, practice at home. Try to facilitate this skill with your child during a time of heightened anxiety, for example, if he gets hurt or calls you into his room in the middle of the night. It is important to practice this routine with your child before a medical event to see if he is comfortable with the coping skill, to determine whether it was effective in helping him get through a difficult situation a little easier.

In helping children cope with a medical procedure, you may be facilitating or engaging them in more than one coping skill simultaneously. Sometimes children will want to use distraction, then move quickly into deep breathing, while also pinching themselves (sensory stimulation), and finding comfort in loved ones' emotional support and undivided attention. Sometimes they will use two or three at the same time. And sometimes a child might use negative coping behaviors, like hitting, biting, or gently pinching himself, yet not doing any actual harm. Remember, however your child copes is OK, as long as he has a less difficult time as a result. Moreover, however your child reacts, you as his parent need to remain calm, soft-spoken, and supportive. Show your child that he is in good hands and can trust his doctor, even though the procedure the doctor is performing may cause discomfort or pain. His perception of the doctor should be positive, and he should understand that the doctor does not want to hurt him, yet some necessary procedures may cause some temporary pain.

Depending on different children's coping styles, two children can be admitted or undergo the same procedure, and the preparation you'd perform would look completely different. To identify your child's style of coping, think of how she has dealt with difficult situations in the past. Make sure to discuss it with her in advance and practice an appropriate technique prior to the procedure, so the child is comfortable and familiar using it. In addition, some children will need to watch the procedure, and others will want to close their eyes or look away. Both ways are acceptable. It is important to note: Let your child make her own choices to better cope with the procedure. Then ensure that you and your child practice this plan repeatedly in advance.

The first coping skill is distraction.

Of the various coping skills, distraction is my favorite because it is what I feel most comfortable doing. It feels most natural to me. Therefore it is easiest for me to walk a child through this and distract them through a time of heightened anxiety or during a procedure. I also utilize this coping technique when I must have a medical procedure myself in which I know I will feel pain. I play music, look at a magazine, or do something to take my mind off what is causing me anxiety or what is scaring me. I have used this technique in many different ways for many different children. It is easy for most parents to find something that will help distract their child. If your child engages in play easily, this will be a very handy tool for you. Get yourself a good picture book, appropriate for your child's age and taste. I use look-and-find books (for example, *Where's Waldo?* or *I Spy*) or books that teach fun and silly facts like *The Way Things Work, Why Is the Sea Salty?* or *Why Do My Eyes Blink?* If your child does not engage in books, you could go out and get a special game for his little handheld game system. The goal is to interact with your child, so pick one that you can participate in, either by asking questions or asking him to show you how to play. Viewfinders, snow globes, and magic wands (sticks with glitter and sequence) work well too.

Save this book or game for doctor visits only, and use these items to create a special interaction between you and your child. You can start distracting when you see the doctors getting ready for a procedure or when your child is getting anxious about a procedure. Show interest in the activity. You can use the popular look-and-find books like *Where's Waldo?* or *Look and Find Scooby Doo* and play a game while searching the book with your child. For example, an effective game is to have a race to find Waldo and keep score of whoever finds Waldo first. Then whoever finds Waldo first gets a point, and the one with the most points gets a prize or reward of some kind.

The appropriate use of positive reinforcement and rewards is taught in greater detail later in the book. Some children really seem to thrive when enticed by a treat or a toy. This technique can easily be used incorrectly or too often, creating a child who will expect rewards consistently. Adding the element of competition can be great for some children but may be difficult for a child who has difficulty with competition or who is a "sore loser." If competition makes your child anxious, the use of this technique may make him more anxious, defeating the purpose of distraction. If this technique seems to keep a child focused longer, however, then utilize this during moments of anxiety. Light competition between parent and child can be a lot of fun for a child, especially when he gets to win.

Let me share an example of a positive interaction I had with a child at the hospital. I was paged to go and prepare a little boy who was going to have a painful procedure. Brayden was 10 years old and needed a spinal tap and bone marrow aspiration. He was simply terrified prior to this procedure. He had suffered through many medical experiences in the past because he had leukemia. I knew him from previous hospitalizations and clinic visits and had an established rapport with him and his mother. Brayden confessed to being afraid of pain and didn't want to be awake for this procedure. Unfortunately, sedation was not an option for him at the time.

So, I prepared him for what he was going to experience, because although he had had this procedure before, this was the first time that he was going to be awake for it. I explained why the doctor needed to do this and why he couldn't have the sedations or "sleepy medicine." I showed him how the procedure would take place. We practiced the position in which the doctor would have him lie, and we tried on the mask the doctor would want him to wear. We went over the procedure, explaining every step in an age-appropriate way. I talked to Brayden about the different ways of coping and asked him which one he wanted to try. He chose to utilize distraction. He wanted to look at a Scooby Doo look-and-find book that I had. Knowing this boy, and knowing that he has had some difficulty coping with painful experiences in the past, I also brought a few other toys and distraction materials with me to his bedside. When the doctor came in, I continued talking to him in a calm and soft voice. I reminded Brayden about his preparation and told him step-by-step what the doctor was doing. When the doctor was ready, this little boy was able to lie on his side, in the position we practiced. To show him that I was advocating for him and understanding his concerns, I conveyed his feelings to the doctor, in front of him. I told the doctor that he was feeling scared and was afraid it was really going to hurt more than he could take. The doctor reassured Brayden he would be as gentle as possible.

Brayden still looked so nervous and seemed interested in what the doctor was doing, watching his every move. I began the distraction exercise once I noticed this behavior. He was able to engage in the exercise until the doctor sat down behind him. Then he began to get upset, so I calmly started talking to him about doing some deep breathing. I asked him to follow me, and I did it with him. This was calming him down, and he picked it up quickly.

As he did his breathing, I began to distract him again. I took out a set of markers, and we began a coloring exercise. He was unable to use his hands so I asked him what marker he would like to use first. He chose green, so I took out the green marker and began to color the mask on his face. I said, "Green? OK. I am going to draw a green nose on your mask." I made a cute smiley face on his mask, then turned the marker to my face. I held it up to my face and told him to guide me in "decorating my mask." He would direct me to where he wanted me to draw and would tell me what to do. We made two eyes, terribly far apart, and a nose above the eyes. Brayden had so much fun in directing me through decorating my mask that we continued this activity until the procedure was over. Once the doctor had cleaned up, we took off our masks; mine was full of funny body parts and pimples. Brayden was laughing and smiling, and he showed no apparent signs of stress or fear. His mother told me that he was a kid who would kick and previously needed to be held down. She was shocked that he could engage in a distraction activity and cope so effectively. Obviously, Brayden trusted me, which enabled me to immerse him in this activity during a time of fear and stress for him.

The second type of coping skill is deep breathing.

As was illustrated in Brayden's story, this is a great skill to use in harmony with any of the other skills, although some children can benefit from this skill all on its own. There are many kinds of deep breathing exercises that a child can do. Breathing exercises have been proven to be very effective for use during times in which an individual experiences intense pain, like during childbirth, when the Lamaze method is often used. There is a simple physiological explanation that helps us understand why breathing exercises, like "Lamaze," work. Physiologically, deep breathing relaxes muscles, increases oxygen supply to the cells, and also encourages the production of endorphins, which are the body's natural pain killers. A parent can easily facilitate a deep breathing exercise with a child by using bubbles or a pinwheel or by pretending to blow out birthday candles. The important part is to teach this skill correctly. This takes practice because a child typically wants to breathe in through her mouth and do it quickly. Teach the child to breathe by taking slow deep breaths in through her nose, deep enough so she can see her tummy fill with air (like watching a balloon fill with air), then slowly release the breath through the mouth with puckered lips (like she is blowing out birthday candles). Once your child understands the skill and can do it effectively, then work on developing a rhythm that remains constant or consistent.

I facilitate this exercise the same way every time to maintain that consistency. First, I accompany the child at her bedside, letting her hold my hand if she chooses. Then I start by modeling this technique. Next we do some practicing, having mom or dad participate. Doing the breathing with the child really helps her stay focused. Here is an example of how you can facilitate this: "OK, let's take a slow deep breath. Now, breathe in through your nose [point to your nose]. Now breathe out through your mouth [point to your mouth]. Again, slowly take a deep breath in through your nose [point to your nose] and out through your mouth [point to the mouth]." I repeat this very same thing over and over until the procedure is finished, maintaining eye contact with the child and keeping the same breathing pattern throughout the entire process.

The third coping skill is guided imagery.

For highly imaginative, serious, and emotional children, this may be the most effective coping skill. I probably utilize this one the least because I have difficulty utilizing this style of coping when I am anxious or scared. In addition, guided imagery is difficult because you need to have a preexisting trusting relationship with the child that will enable her to trust in you enough to be "guided."

As a parent, it is important to recognize that the use of guided imagery will only work if you have already established an open and trusting relationship with your child, specifically in regard to her medical situation. In the next chapter, we will discuss how to make sure you and your child have this kind of relationship. Often parents assume that they have their child's trust and do not realize how easy it is for a child to lose this trust from a simple lie, hidden truth, or misunderstanding. A trusting relationship is essential and will need to be established or reestablished. This is done through consistency, truth, advocacy, and empathy. Once you reestablish this trust, your child will close her eyes for this technique and let you guide her into an imaginative experience.

To determine whether your child is able to engage in guided imagery, ask your child to practice at home. See if your child is comfortable doing this and if she gets into it. If she is easily distracted or cannot keep her eyes closed, this is probably not the coping skill of choice for your child. If she is capable of closing her eyes doing this at home, practice it, because it is more difficult to completely engage her during times when she is afraid. Keep in mind that this technique requires someone she trusts to guide an imaginary experience.

An example of a guided imagery experience is using the imagination to go on a pretend trip to a favorite place. Many children pick the beach, the park, or Disneyland. You guide their experience to this place in their imagination. They close their eyes and picture the place. The facilitator would focus the child's attention on different sensory aspects of this place. For example, if you want to take a trip to the beach, you ask the child to close her eyes and imagine being at the beach. You ask questions about who is with her, and challenge her to see who is there and why they came along. Then you could ask the child what everyone is wearing and to describe their outfits and bathing suits. You could ask what the weather is like, and ask the child to try to feel the cold ocean water rushing over her feet or the sand squishing between her toes. Some children are food lovers; have the child describe what is in her picnic basket and what everything tastes like. The key is to engage the child so deeply that she forgets she is undergoing a procedure. When I was first getting started as a Child Life Specialist, I was skeptical about the success of this activity until I saw it work with patients time and time again.

The last coping skill is seeking sensory stimulation.

This is not the kind of coping skill that you teach to children. You wouldn't want to choose this skill as a means to cope if you can introduce the others first. Children who have not had the benefit of someone with the right tools helping them through a scary time tend to either have already developed a negative coping skill or will prefer to cope using sensory stimulation. These kids do things like hit, pinch, or bite themselves to decrease the feelings of pain felt during a procedure like a needle poke. Although this may not be ideal, there is a physiological explanation for it. When multiple sensory receptors are stimulated at the same time, the message that is sent to the brain telling us to feel pain is confused or diminished. Pain that is self-administered, like pinching yourself, can disperse the feelings of pain between two locations, typically making the needle pain feel much less painful.

I was once paged by a nurse to come and assist her in giving Connor an IV, in the Pediatric Intensive Care Unit (PICU) of our hospital. He was five years old and definitely an "avoider". Connor had a chronic illness that required many admissions to the hospital and unfortunately many needle pokes and painful procedures over his lifetime. As a result, he had established a coping style that worked for him but was not easily accepted by his parents or the nursing staff. He never wanted information from the nurses and avoided eye contact with them when they approached. Connor would cope by seeking sensory stimulation and would achieve this by repeatedly smacking himself on the side of the head. It was unpleasant to watch, but this coping skill enabled him to endure yet another poke.

The nurses called me and asked me to work on getting him to try something else to help him cope. I was unable to get him to engage in a less intrusive coping skill; he was simply not going for it. Connor's parents were yelling at him to stop. The nurses were uncomfortable with a child hitting himself repeatedly, yet Connor persisted. Once the nurses reached for the "hitting hand," he began to scream, and his anxiety level skyrocketed. He began to flop and flail about the bed and was inconsolable. This is when I asked the nurses to stop and give Connor a break. We discussed the procedure and identified that this was the only way for him to cope with the IV, so I educated the nurses, discussed this with his parents, and facilitated this coping during his IV. To reiterate, this is not a coping skill that I would teach or encourage a child to use, but the point is, this is what helped him; it is what he needed to soothe himself. As long as he was not putting himself in danger, my job was to help him cope, even if that meant enabling him to hit himself during a procedure.

No matter which coping skill you and your child decide to use, it is important for you to remain calm when facilitating this experience for your child. Your child reacts to your affect, whether she means to or not. If you are anxious, your child will be too. I like to tell parents to put this to the test: If your child is loud and crying, be calm and quiet. Get close to her, hug or hold her, and stroke her hair. Speak slowly and quietly, taking long deep breaths for her to see and hear. Breathe in through your nose and out through your mouth. It is amazing how much quicker the child will calm down and move toward your level. It is much more calming and soothing for her, so she will typically respond more favorably than if you were talking fast or loud, thinking that you needed to talk over her crying or screaming. Ultimately, anxiety feeds off of anxiety, and the crying will continue for a longer period of time.

Chapter 2 Review

1. *Introduce coping skills to your child to assist him in times of heightened anxiety or difficult life situations.*

2. *Children usually are either avoiders or information seekers when it comes to medical knowledge. Information seekers want information; avoiders typically do not.*

3. *The four major coping skills are distraction, deep breathing, guided imagery, and seeking sensory stimulation.*

A Strong Tower of Trust: Fostering a Trusting Relationship with Your Child

Jaime

Jaime is a little girl who had to have tubes put into her ears because she had seven ear infections in her two short years of life. She had been to the doctor before, and her mom tries to make her experiences with her doctor positive and holds the doctor in a positive light. Jaime's mom has taught her that the doctor helps her and wants to make sure that her body grows up the right way. Therefore, Jaime likes her doctor and plays doctor at home frequently. She always speaks of him fondly and tells her Fisher-Price patients, "You have owie? It's OK. Doctor is going to fix it."

Recently, Jaime had immunizations and blood work done. She calls these shots and lab draws "pokies." She, like everyone else on the planet, doesn't like pokies. Nevertheless, Jaime's mother told her one morning that they had to go to the doctor that day and told her that the doctor had to do a pokie to test her blood. Jaime got a very worried little look on her face. Her eyes welled up with tears as she said, "I don't want to get a pokie." Her mom picked her up and comforted her and said, "I know, honey. I wouldn't want to get a pokie either. Pokies hurt, don't they? Remember, honey, that it only hurts for a short time, and Mommy is going to be with you the whole time. I can hold your hand if you want, or I can rub your back. You tell me what you want me to do to help you. Once the nurse gets what she needs, you will be all done. Then there will be no more pokies. Then Mommy will take you home, and you won't need another pokie for a long time."

In the waiting room, Jaime was pacing, back and forth, back and forth, climbing from chair to chair. She knew her time was coming, and her mom could tell she was nervous. Jaime's mom brought some comfort items from home for when they called Jaime into the lab. She brought Jaime's special blankie and her pacifier to help her cope with this pokie. When the lab technician called Jaime's name, she ran to her mom's arms, clearly nervous and afraid. Her mom reminded her that it would only hurt for a moment and that "Mommy would be there with her the whole time." Her mom held her close and spoke softly into Jaime's ear, telling her how much she loved her and what an amazing girl she was. By providing her comfort and a pacifier, Jaime got through this pokie without screaming or crying. As a matter of fact, she did not make one peep. But her brow remained furrowed and her eyes gazed around inquisitively until she left the lab. The key to this successful coping experience was that she had a coping mechanism (sucking on the pacifier) and she absolutely trusted her mom, which allowed her to trust the environment and the phlebotomist.

Sometime later, Jaime went to the pre-op appointment for the tubes surgery. When her mom told her that the doctor she was going to meet was a new doctor who was going to look into her ears to see if there was something she could do to help her ears not hurt her anymore, Jaime displayed a few signs of concern. She wanted her mom to hold her a lot and continued to protest. She cried and said that she didn't want to go. Her mom addressed her behavior by saying, "I see that you feel scared to go to the doctor. But we still have to go. This doctor is nice, and she is only going to look into your ears. No pokies." Jaime's concerns were diminished, and she went into the doctor's office without hesitation. She knew that her mom was telling her the truth and she had nothing to fear.

Many children and adults perceive the hospital experience negatively or as a punishment. I cannot tell you how many times during my career I have heard parents use the doctor and shots or needles as a threat to make a screaming or crying child stop or to try to get a child to "behave." When parents threaten a child with a needle, they completely destroy their child's view of the doctor. By teaching the child that a doctor enforces punishment, they ruin their child's perception that the doctor is there to help him. In addition, this diminishes the parent's role as the child's authority figure. With a negative view of doctors (whom they will have to visit regularly throughout their lifetime), children grow up with negative feelings about medical experiences that evoke fear and anxiety in all medical situations. These traumatized patients usually grow up to be fearful adults because once they are traumatized by the medical environment, it is very difficult to turn their feelings into positive ones later in life.

A trusting relationship is essential for children to get through the medical experience without stress and trauma that will last into adulthood. So many parents cover up the truth, mislead their children, or withhold information about medical situations. As a result, there are many children who do not trust their parents in the medical arena. If your child does not believe you when you tell him that he is not going to get a shot or if he cries and resists even when you tell him that measuring his height does not hurt, he does not feel he can trust you. This does not mean that you have a bad relationship with your child. Nor does it mean that you do not have a trusting relationship outside of the medical arena. Importantly, it does not mean that you are a bad parent!

The fact is that all of us make mistakes while having our child's best interests in mind. If you are reading this book, you have your child's best interests in mind! Unfortunately, that does not change the fact that you could have lied to your child in the past to try and prevent him from crying or being afraid about a doctor's visit or a trip to the hospital. It's possible that you didn't know you were lying or that it wasn't a good idea. However, if this is the case, your child will most likely find it hard to believe you when discussing what really is going on with him medically and cannot trust that you are being totally honest with him about his medical experiences. If this sounds familiar, your child will need someone else to rely on, temporarily, until you can rebuild that trust. This "trusting person" can be a family member or a friend. Sometimes a medical professional can act as a child's "trusting person" if the parent/child relationship is not yet nurturing and trusting. This is usually the role of the Child Life Specialist or a favorite nurse.

Establishing or reestablishing a trusting relationship with your child is easier than it seems.

To maintain this trust, you must be forthright at all times. You must not mislead your child, withhold information, or get caught in a lie. For example, your child might ask you, "Is it going to hurt, Mommy?" If you say, "No, honey, it's not going to hurt," and it actually does hurt, the child experiences what I call "unexpected pain." The trust you have built with your child is ruined. This makes future experiences very frustrating and unpredictable for the child. He will not know what to expect or whom to trust, and he will know he cannot trust you, the person he looks to for comfort and answers. The next time he has a medical question, he will not ask you and will typically be afraid even when the doctors or nurses perform non-invasive procedures, such as taking a temperature and measuring blood pressure, because he fears unexpected pain.

Instead, to foster a trusting relationship you could say, "Yes, honey, it is going to hurt. It is going to feel like you are being pinched. It only lasts for a short time, and I am going to be there with you the whole time. I can hold your hand if you want. We can bring your bubbles or your *Where's Waldo?* book to look at. I asked the doctor, and he said that you would only have one poke. I know you are scared (or mad), but you are going to be OK. It is OK to cry, and it is OK to be scared. I would be scared too. Do you have any questions or worries, honey?" It may seem difficult to be honest all the time, but simple truth is essential and must be maintained or you will end up right back where you started.

In the scenario just described, you are being honest with your child and preparing him by addressing sensory concerns. You are telling the child that you are there to help him and are giving him some control (by letting him choose your level of involvement). You are also offering him a coping skill (bubbles or book), are validating your child's feelings, and are reassuring him that he is going to be OK. Then, importantly, you are providing your child an option to ask questions or express his concerns in a safe environment. All of that explained in only 10 sentences nurtures your relationship with your child. *You can do this!*

To further reestablish this trusting relationship, you can follow a simple five-step approach to building better trust. The five steps are:

1. Admit

2. Address

3. Reassure

4. Check in

5. Remind.

First, explain to your child that you are trying to be more open with her and are trying to help her better understand what is happening in her medical situation. Make an effort to translate medical lingo or jargon into an age-appropriate language that your child will understand. It is important that you acknowledge prior situations in which you were not totally honest with your child. Let her know that you thought you were doing the right thing by trying to minimize the situation or hide the truth because you didn't want to see her scared and didn't want her to cry. Tell your child that you thought you were making it easier for her. This leads to the first step in the process.

ADMIT that these tactics were not the best way to help her cope. Then offer your child an apology and plenty of hugs.

Next, **ADDRESS** the fact that you know she may have lost trust in you. You could do this by asking your child, "Do you worry that I am not going to tell you the truth?" or "Are you afraid that Mommy isn't telling you everything?"

Then, **REASSURE** your child that you are going to be honest about the doctor and medical procedures from now on.

Periodically **CHECK IN** with your child by asking her, "How are you feeling about how I described how the procedure would go?" or "Did I do a good job telling you everything the doctor was going to do?"

REMIND your child that you are doing your best to accurately inform her about all medical events and procedures and are committed to building a more trusting relationship. Last, stick to it! Repeat these steps on a routine basis. This should greatly improve your relationship with your child, and you should see a reduction in anxiety at the doctor's office.

If you find yourself stuck or unable to answer your child's question appropriately, then tell her you are not sure of the answer, but that you will ask the doctor or the nurse for her. This is a great time to make use of that small notebook or journal that was discussed in Chapter 1. This journal can be taken to the doctor with you to make sure that all of your child's questions have been addressed, which means fulfilling your commitment to her and helping her understand her medical situation. Your child will benefit in the long run. She will be more trusting of you in all situations, will cope better with anxiety, and will learn that she can rely on you and others for support.

This does not mean that your child will have no anxiety whatsoever. Children are going to have anxiety about painful events. But the knowledge that they have someone who loves them and somcone they trust with them allows them to better cope with their anxiety and reduce the stress and trauma caused by uncertainty and unknowing. With information and trust, a child's anxiety is going to be much easier to deflate with the help of reassurance and the teaching of coping skills.

Chapter 3 Review

1. *Children need a trusting relationship that will enable them to open their minds to being taught to use coping skills during times of heightened anxiety.*

2. *Establishing or reestablishing a trusting relationship is easier than you think.*

3. *The five steps to developing a trusting relationship are: Admit, Address, Reassure, Check in, and Remind.*

Chapter 4

Children Need to Feel Understood

Gregory

In a medical setting, the majority of children (and adults) have anxiety, fear, and a ton of questions needing answers. From my experience, I have noticed that parents try to diffuse these feelings in their children instead of addressing them. As a result, children feel frustrated, ignored, and misunderstood, and they oftentimes display signs of anger and resentment toward their parents. Why is this? Well, let's think this through as a child would. It is important to remember that children move through stages of development. Their brains become more complex and develop logical thinking by about age 7. But it is important to note that most children regress, meaning they temporarily move backward in their development, when faced with a foreign and/or difficult situation like the hospital or a medical procedure. So one could argue that even older school-age children lack the skills and cognitive development necessary to make sense of and make peace with the medical environment without assistance from an empathetic caregiver. Typically, most children would rationalize this way, "My parent drove me to this scary place, made me come here, and see the doctor. When I cried, I got yelled at. Then, my parent sat back and watched and allowed the scary nurses to hurt me." They wonder, "Why are you mad at me? What did I do wrong? Why am I being punished?"

Knowing and understanding that this is a typical child's reaction to the medical environment makes it easier for adults to understand why the hospital and the doctor pose such a threat to children. It makes it easier to see that their behaviors—such as tantrums, kicking, screaming, crying, and meltdowns—are typically fearful reactions rather than "bad behavior." Being mindful of this is key to being able to give your child the empathetic, nurturing support he needs in the medical environment, even when his behavior is such that you want to get angry at him or discipline him.

To clarify this point, I am going to introduce you to a boy named Gregory. Gregory was four years old when I met him and midway through his cancer treatments. Gregory was a difficult patient because he did not trust anyone. He was afraid of the simplest procedure. He required being held down for most of his routine care and had to be bargained with so he would take his oral medicines. The nurses had to come in when he was asleep to start his IV meds and his chemotherapy, or cancer medicine.

His mom was a very nice lady and seemed to have a very good relationship with her son. She was at his bedside all the time and provided him with toys and distraction activities. They played together by the bedside all the time. At first, it was hard to figure out why Gregory had such poor coping skills. Then I found out what was going on at home.

Gregory's condition called for him to come to the outpatient clinic two times a week and to be admitted to the hospital frequently for chemotherapy. All the while, he was never told for what reason he was coming to the hospital. His mom didn't want to use the word "cancer" in front of him. She told him that he was just "sick." His visits to the doctor were difficult, but he got used to going and developed a relationship with one nurse that he seemed to be a trusting relationship. He asked for her every time, and she was the only one who could get him to take his oral meds and was the only nurse he would let touch him without putting up a fight.

It was from this caring nurse that I learned how his mom was having a great amount of difficulty getting him to agree to come to these appointments and to the hospital. This kind nurse sought help because she felt that this family needed help but was unsure how to approach the subject with Gregory's mother. It is easy for us to see that his fear stemmed from hidden truths and misconceptions that he formed due to a lack of knowledge and lack of emotional support from his mother. In trying to protect him from the truth, she actually caused him more pain without realizing it.

When they next came to the hospital, I made a plan to speak to Gregory's mom; I hoped to help her see the root cause of Gregory's outward behaviors. She wanted to help her son and wanted him to be unafraid. It seemed that she was mostly concerned about controlling his "bad" behavior. She rationalized her decision to keep Gregory's diagnosis from him, and in the end, she sadly stood her ground and kept up the lie. My involvement in Gregory's case was limited to providing toys for distraction and taking him to the playroom to offer him some normalcy in the hospital.

Cases like this are difficult for me to accept. Sometimes parents have different cultural values and belief systems that cause them to resist the help that I have to offer. In fact, the initial reason that I started this book is because of my feelings of sadness for these children and the helplessness I felt as I was crippled in helping them.

A child must know that his parent is on his side in order to provide him with comfort and trust, which are necessary for him to be able to positively cope with his environment. This goes for life situations as well, not just medical situations. Children need to know that their parent is an advocate for them, someone who will help them through their experiences and help them get their needs met by helping them communicate their feelings, fears, and concerns when they are unable to do so. They find comfort and assurance in a parent who will listen or identify what they are concerned about and show understanding, even if their feelings seem silly, invalid, or "childish." Children, like adults, want someone to validate their feelings. In addition, children need someone to help them make sense of their feelings and identify them and to provide comfort, assurance, and direction.

In some cases, this means talking to the doctor to help a child get his needs met. In many cases, the parent is the expert in this, but for some reason, when moms and dads enter the medical environment, they feel at the liberty of that nurse or doctor. Many are afraid to ask for what they want and usually will not question the methods of the nurse or doctor. As an advocate for your child, you must do exactly that. If there is something you or your child is uncomfortable with in the medical environment, you need to address the situation and take control. This could be a number of things. You could want or need a translator, a better explanation of a procedure or diagnosis, a different product or medicine, a different nurse, a different bed or room, to speak to the doctor again, and so forth. Whatever it is, in seeking more information and advocating for your child's needs and wishes, you are showing your child that you care and that you are there to help him through a difficult time.

A parent who advocates for his or her child makes sure that the medical staff is aware of the child's fear of needles and asks for a topical anesthetic. An advocate would convey the child's fear to the nurse who is about to remove the tape from a wound, requesting and getting adhesive remover if it would make it easier for the child. When a child sees his parent doing this, it helps the child understand that his parent is addressing his concerns and understands what he is feeling. It is such a relief for children to know that their mom or dad is listening to their fears and concerns and helping them cope with their situation. Children need to be heard just like adults do. It is important for them to know that you are on their team and that their feelings are understood, whether you agree with them or not. They need adults to identify and label feelings for them and help them make sense of new feelings that arise when confronted with medical situations.

A well-known pediatrician named Harvey Karp, who is a professor and doctor at UCLA, has written a few excellent books that I have used in rearing my children. One is called *The Happiest Baby on the Block*, a book that provides strategies to evoke a calming reflex in a baby. He introduces "The Five S's," which elicit this calming reflex and can turn a crying, screaming baby into a calm and comforted one. His idea is that if parents help mimic the womb for a newborn, almost providing the infant with a "fourth trimester," the child will feel more relaxed, nurtured, and comforted.

Dr. Karp's second book is called *The Happiest Toddler on the Block*, in which he boldly states that children who are not yet able to communicate linguistically are like cavemen. They babble and have "o" and "ah" sounds that they use to communicate a want or need. Dr. Karp says that you need to be like an ambassador for your children, showing them how to communicate and helping them make sense of their surroundings. This is how you teach your children to communicate more effectively. In doing so, you must show your children that you understand what they are trying to communicate and label their feelings and emotions for them, like an ambassador.

Dr. Karp also teaches that, when a toddler is having a tantrum, a parent can mimic the tantrum while crying, "You want. You want the cookie. Jake wants the cookie. He wants to eat the cookie because cookies are yummy." It is when the toddler realizes that you get it, when he feels understood, that the tantrum stops. My kids would actually stop the tantrum and start to laugh. They would look at me like, "What are you doing?" The amazing thing is that the tantrum stops. Why? Because you understood what your child was trying to tell you and you showed him that you understood. Having your child calmed down and able to listen, you are then able to say something supportive, respectful, and clear like, "I hear you, honey. You want the cookie. You can have one after dinner. Let's go play with your dollhouse." This works effectively with the toddlers, my own and the little ones I have worked with. Many times I have stopped a tantrum using this brilliant principle. It is amazing to me that once the child feels that a grown-up understands his want or need, he feels validated and much less frustrated, and tantrums tend to cease before they get out of hand.

Feeling understood is feeling respected. When a child feels respected, he has a higher self-esteem and has an easier time developing trusting relationships. These early lasting relationships are the building blocks for future relationships throughout life.

Chapter 4 Review

1. *Children need to feel that their parents truly understand their feelings about being sick or in the hospital.*

2. *Parents need to act as an advocate for their child.*

3. *Parents need to provide their child with empathy and understanding, even when the child's behaviors do not seem appropriate.*

4. *Spend time talking with children about medical events simply and truthfully.*

Developmentally Appropriate Education and Communication

Jonathan

Too many children go through medical events without any knowledge of what is to come. In my experience, much of a child's fear stems from misconception and misunderstanding. Hospitals and most medical environments are totally foreign to children. Although many children have been to the doctor's office on multiple occasions, the medical environment is different than any other place that children have been, and every time they go to this setting, their experiences are different. It is not only a foreign place; it is also an unpredictable place. Medical professionals have their own language using strange words and abbreviations, spoken like a secret code. Medical jargon leaves many adults confused and feeling frustrated, so just imagine how confusing and frustrating this is for children—especially when they are not given the opportunity to ask questions or express themselves.

This is a simple yet complicated phenomenon. Children need to know what is going on! They need to be told, step-by-step, what is going to happen to them to alleviate fear of the unknown and to avoid misconception. That seems easy enough, doesn't it? However, if parents cannot effectively prepare their child because their own understanding is unclear, how is a child supposed to cope with this uncertain and unpredictable situation? In the best cases, a medical center or doctor's office has a professional who provides age-appropriate preparation for families. When this is not available, however, it is up to a parent or caregiver to assume this role. This may seem difficult; sometimes parents don't fully understand the medical event themselves. So how are they supposed to prepare their children? *Call the doctor.* Ask him or her questions. If the doctor is unavailable, ask questions at the pre-op appointment or ask the nurse. Make sure you will be able to address the following concerns/questions for your child:

- Who (Who will the child see?)

- What (What are they going to do to the child?)

- When (When is the surgery, and how long will it hurt?)

- Where (Where will the child be, and where will the parent be?)

- Why (Why is this happening to the child? Did the child do something wrong?)

Definitely ensure that you ask the doctor or a medical professional associated with the particular procedure questions that address a child's sensory experiences. Ask the doctor what the child will be feeling, seeing, hearing, and smelling; then explain all this to your child in a safe environment. For some children this can be done during play; for others it is best done at a favorite place or over an ice cream. Make sure your child feels at ease, safe, and supported during any potentially threatening conversations.

I want to tell you the story of a child named Jonathan. Jonathan was in the hospital after an appendectomy, a surgery in which the appendix is removed. Typically, a child who has had an uncomplicated appendectomy is admitted to the hospital for a short time so doctors can manage his pain and make sure he is able to eat, drink, pee, and poop without complication. Then the child is discharged home. Sometimes the child goes home the day of the surgery. Jonathan was ready to be discharged, but the discharge was held up because he wasn't eating. He refused and wouldn't tell anyone why. I was asked to come and see this patient. Because the doctors did not find a medical reason for his hunger strike, they assumed he had something else going on.

After a long introduction, over a game of Chutes and Ladders, he finally started talking to me. I told him what my job was, and I asked him if I could teach him about the surgery he just had. He was hesitant, but he said yes. After our game was over, I went to get an anatomy doll that I use to teach children about their bodies. I explained what his surgery was and showed him what the surgeon removed while focusing on issues that I knew would concern an eight-year-old. I explained to Jonathan that the doctor removed a part of his body that he didn't need. I explained that there is no use for an appendix and that his body was not going to miss his appendix. I also showed him where the appendix was in the body using my anatomy doll.

After explaining this to Jonathan, I saw instant relief on his face. He began to make and hold eye contact with me, so I asked him if he had any questions about his operation. He looked like he did, but didn't ask. Then I explained that there was nothing he did that caused his appendix to become infected and need to be removed. I told him that it was not his fault and that this particular infection happens to a lot of boys his age. We continued to talk a bit more, and then he finally revealed, "I ate too many Flaming Hot Cheetos. My mom told me that if I ate too many, my stomach would hurt, so the doctors took it out." Ultimately, Jonathan associated the pain he experienced from the infection with eating too many chips. Once I was able to convince him that Flaming Hot Cheetos were not the cause of his appendicitis and that his stomach and appendix were two different parts of the body (illustrating this on the anatomy doll), he began to eat again and went home that evening.

Jonathan spent two days feeling terrified. Not only did he think that he was completely to blame for his hospitalization, he was also afraid to tell anyone because he thought he would be punished for eating the Cheetos. In addition, he had formed a misconception and thought that the doctors removed his stomach! This was the reason he was afraid to eat. If this little boy had been prepared appropriately, he would have been able to go home a day or two earlier because his fears and misconceptions would not have prevented him from recovering.

Many children have similar experiences, in which they are never appropriately prepared for procedures or surgeries. They will seek or avoid information. Furthermore, the information they get is usually not presented to them, but to their parents. Therefore, the children are not getting developmentally appropriate explanations, which is one of the reasons for the misconceptions. This problem is very common in children who need to undergo medical procedures or surgery. They take the information they hear the doctors giving their parents, combine that with information they've learned from television or the experiences of friends and family, and form a very detailed misconception about their medical situation. Usually, the misconceptions they form are far more traumatic and scary than the actual situations.

You can now see why it is essential for you to effectively communicate with your child about medical events. It is also important for you to have some knowledge of the psychological development of children and the effects of illness, hospitalization, and the medical environment on a child. Medical events will affect children differently depending on their level of development and their family situation. Although it is important to remember that within every developmental level each child is unique and will react individually, these general concepts cover some of the issues that children and their families may face when the child requires medical intervention.

Consider the following developmental needs before preparing your child for a medical experience.

Basic Needs of Developmental Stages

Infants need:

- Predictable, trusting relationship

- Sensory (verbal, auditory, visual, and tactile) stimulation, without over stimulating

- Soothing and comforting by parental presence and by providing pleasurable stimuli (holding, touching, rocking)

- Consistency and stability in care (establish nap time and feeding routines)

Toddlers need:

- A trusting relationship with parents

- Physical space to explore and practice using gross motor (large muscles) movements such as jumping, skipping, spinning in a circle, climbing

- Several opportunities to play

- Consistency, stability, and predictability found in a daily routine

- Parental acceptance of regression under stress

- Special security objects like blankets, pacifiers, teddy bears

- Opportunity to gain independence

- Positive reinforcement and reassurance during procedures or treatments

- Cuddling and hugging from parents

- Simple and repeated explanations about medical events

Preschool children need:

- Their feelings identified for them (that is, "I see that you are feeling very frustrated when the doctor talks to me. Do you feel like we are ignoring you?")

- Opportunity for play or to express themselves through art and music

- Consistency, stability, and predictability found in daily routines (nap, meals, and play)

- Repetitious explanations about procedures and events

- Familiar toys and security objects to help them cope

- To be offered choices whenever possible

- Stability in parenting (biting, hitting, kicking, or aggressive behaviors toward others are still unacceptable behaviors when a child is sick and/or hospitalized)

- To be taught acceptable expression of angry feelings (talking, art, or pounding something safe like a pillow or couch)

- Rewards for good behavior and coping with procedure or tests

School-age children need:

- Involvement and play time with peers

- Parental presence during interactions with doctors and medical staff

- Opportunities to play and express themselves through art and music

- Explanations they are able to understand about procedures, tests, diagnosis, and treatment plan

- Teachings about feelings and how to manage feelings of fear and anxiety

- Opportunity to make choices regarding their care (when possible)

- Reassurance that feelings of sadness, anger, and guilt are normal

- Consoling about missed activities (school, sports, friends)

- Daily physical activity

Adolescents need:

- Recognition of concerns about body image and need for privacy

- Continuation of normal activities like schooling, music, computer, texting, sports

- Detailed preparation and explanations

- Involvement in all discussions about their care

- Opportunity to talk privately with medical professionals and with peers

- Parental involvement when necessary or requested

- Opportunities for increasing independence and responsibility

- Understanding from parents if the child regresses during times of heightened anxiety

- Comfort and empathy

- Encouragement for teens to share feelings and thoughts with peers (phone calls, email, chats, and texts)

Once parents are able to identify what their child needs to cope effectively with medical situations, communicating with the child is of great importance. You have to choose your words carefully, giving just the right amount of information with care in using safe, non-threatening words. Children of all ages benefit from communication that is honest, simple, and given to them out of love. Here are some tips about communicating with a child:

Communication Tips for Parents and Caregivers

✓ Be clear and consistent in parenting. If, for example, hitting is not OK at home, it is not acceptable at the doctor's office either. Mean what you say. This gives children predictability and stability.

✓ Tell the child what is appropriate and inappropriate behavior. "It is OK to cry if you are hurt or afraid." Or, "It is not OK for you to hit and kick because you are scared or angry."

✓ Speak *only* truth. If you do not know the answers to the child's questions, be honest about it. Say, "I don't know, but that is a good question, and we will ask the doctor as soon as we see him."

✓ *Be honest* when your child asks, "Will it hurt?" Explain as best you can what it will feel like. I like using the words "pinch" or "poke." Avoid using threatening words like "bee sting," "puppy bite," "stick," or "prick."

✓ Recognize when your child is trying to express a feeling or tell you about a concern. Then repeat it back to the child, putting what you have heard him say into your own words. Help the child figure out a way for his wishes to be understood or his concerns addressed. This shows your child that you are listening and understanding his feelings and communicates to him that you are on his team.

✓ Help the child express feelings by allowing him time to play, role play, or express himself however he is most comfortable. Some children do this through art, music, journaling, or talking with friends.

✓ Validate your child's feelings. "It is OK to be afraid. I will be here with you the whole time" or "I see you are feeling mad. It is OK to be mad; do you want to hit this pillow?" Remember, tantrums are developmentally appropriate reactions for toddlers, and crying is a normal reaction for children of all ages.

✓ Offer choices when possible. "It seems that you are angry because you have to take this medicine. It is OK to be angry and to dislike your medicine, but you must take it to help you get better. Do you want to take it before or after this TV show?"

✓ If a child does not have a choice about a given situation, do not give one. Instead, give the child direction that tells him what to do: "It is time to take your medicine." **Do not say,** "Do you want to take your medicine now?" By asking a question, you are giving the child control over the situation, but then taking it away. A child sees this as exerting authority.

✓ Give your child positive suggestions rather than commands: "Why don't you try sitting up for awhile? I am concerned about your body getting weak and tired if you don't exercise it." This is much better than, "You need to get up and walk. You need your exercise."

In an ideal situation, a parent or medical professional would prepare your child before surgery. Here is an example of a way to prepare a school-age child for an appendectomy:

✓ *You are having a surgery to take out your appendix because your appendix is infected and because it hurts you. You did not do anything to cause your appendix to get infected. Many children have surgeries to take out their appendix too.*

✓ *The surgery you are having is called an "appendectomy." This means the doctor will have to take your appendix out. The appendix doesn't do anything for your body, but sometimes it gets swollen and causes pain. The pain will not go away until the appendix comes out.*

✓ *The doctor always does surgery in a very special place called an operating room. It is special because it is super clean, probably the cleanest place in the world. It is so clean that there are no germs in it. Only specially cleaned people with specially cleaned outfits are allowed to go into the operating room. This is to make sure that your body is safe from getting a different kind of infection.*

✓ *You will know you are in the operating room when you see big round lights that hang from the ceiling.*

✓ *The doctor and the nurses all will be wearing specially cleaned clothes; sometimes they are green and sometimes they are blue. They wear hats on their head to cover their hair. They also wear a mask to cover their mouth and their nose, so they don't breathe any germs into the operating room. [Many doctor's offices have these items or something similar; ask for them so you can take them home to use to prepare your child.]*

✓ *The doctors will give you a special sleepy medicine, called anesthesia. It will make you go to sleep for just enough time for them to complete your surgery. You will not wake up during your surgery. You will wake up after your surgery is over.*

✓ *The anesthesia will make your body sleep so you don't have to do it by yourself. It also makes your mind sleep so you won't remember anything.*

✓ *Remember, you will not feel anything during your surgery. You will be sleeping the whole time.*

✓ *Once you are asleep, the doctor will make a small opening right here [showing where the incision will be, below your belly button but above the pelvic bone] to take the appendix out. Remember, you will be asleep when he does this, so you won't feel anything.*

✓ *Once the doctor takes the appendix out, he closes the opening he made with a special tape or glue that is only for skin.*

✓ *While the doctor is doing the surgery, your mom or dad will be waiting right outside the doors.*

You will get to see him or her right after you wake up.

✓ *Once you are awake, you will feel that there is some tape or a bandage below your belly button. This is to keep your opening clean and help it heal faster.*

✓ *Most kids say that after their surgery is over, they feel sore, and the muscles around their belly hurt for a couple of days. The doctors and nurses will give you medicine, like Tylenol, that will help make the pain go away.*

✓ *You will not miss your appendix. Once your body heals from this surgery, you won't feel any different. In fact, you probably won't even know that it's gone.*

✓ *It usually takes about a week or two for you to feel totally better. When you do, you will be able to do everything you are used to doing, like playing soccer, swimming, and riding your bike, and you will have a very cool story to tell your friends when you get home.*

This is one way to prepare an older child about her surgery. For a younger child, you would keep the focus on sensory experiences with less detail about the doctor and processes. A younger child would need more reassurance that you are going to be there when she wakes up and need to be prepared for the "owie" when she wakes up.

Everyone has an individual style and ways of explaining the surgical process. I believe that if you can explain surgery as a step-by-step process, while addressing sensory information, you give the child a clear picture of what she is going to be experiencing. That way she is "prepared" and will not experience anything unpredictable that may frighten her. A preparation like this can be explained all in one sitting or it can be broken up and the child prepared in stages if she is unable or unwilling to listen through the explanation's entirety.

It is important that you make sure to let the child guide the preparation. If she does not want to hear the information, don't force her. Allow her to ask questions; remember, answer as best you can without compromising the truth! It's OK not to know the answer. It's not OK to mislead or lie to the child.

Chapter 5 Review

1. *Children need age-appropriate education about their medical diagnosis and about any procedures, both invasive and non-invasive.*

2. *Parents need to act as advocate for their child, obtaining the appropriate information from the doctor's office and translating it into information that is appropriate for the child's level of understanding.*

3. *Tell children step-by-step what is going to happen to them to alleviate their fear of the unknown and to avoid misconceptions.*

4. *Spend time talking with children about medical events in an environment that feels safe for them. Always speak simply and truthfully.*

Step-by-Step Preparation for Their Experiences

Amy

One of the first patients I ever accompanied to a procedure was a child who was going for a spinal tap. She was six years old and had cancer. She was in her second month of treatment, and I was brand-new to the hospital. She had a spinal tap before and had great difficulty coping with the pain. To me this was a challenge that felt more like mission impossible. I was unsure that I could help an already scared and traumatized child.

Her name was Amy. She sat in the waiting room, crying for about an hour before I got to see her. Her parents said that she was really afraid and typically was a very shy and timid little girl who did not cope well with pain or anxiety- evoking situations. I brought a teaching doll and medical play equipment. I talked to her about the procedure and what she remembered from the previous time. While we played with my doll, I talked to her about why the doctor needed to do the procedure. She got to watch me perform a pretend spinal tap on the doll, and then she got to try it. She liked this activity and repeated the spinal tap on the doll many times until the doctor called her to the procedure room. At this point, she began to cry and got very anxious. She refused to go, which embarrassed her parents. Her father reacted by picking her up and carrying her into the procedure room kicking and screaming.

Once we got in the room and saw the doctor and two nurses, Amy's fear escalated. In this small procedure room were two nurses, one doctor, the two parents, and me, the Child Life Specialist. Six adults were hovering over her single little body, which was being held down on the table. Ideally, a child would be comfortable enough to curl up in an suitable position for the doctor so she wouldn't have to be held. And if she was too afraid and unable to hold her body still, she would know in advance that the nurses were going to help her hold still. This way, the child's perception would still be positive, having assistance from the nurses as opposed to being pinned down by a big person. Imagine for a minute the feeling of being held down by someone bigger and stronger than you. How terrifying is this feeling for any of us?

It wasn't long before I noticed that all five other adults were talking to Amy, shouting over each other to be heard. Her parents were trying to correct her behavior, threatening that she wouldn't get to go home if she didn't cooperate. The nurses were talking loudly to get her to hold still, and the doctor was frustrated and telling her to stop moving. When Amy couldn't do this, the nurses restrained her so the doctor could begin his procedure. I bent down, locked eyes with her, and began to talk softly. I could see her trying to focus her attention on my words, tuning out the rest of the adults talking to her. I began to facilitate a deep breathing exercise with Amy, and through her tears and screaming, she was able to do the breathing pretty well. What I found most interesting was that, in the moment of heightened anxiety, she immediately picked up a calm and nurturing tone in my voice and affect and sought to come down to my level. Amy tuned out her parents and the doctor and chose to listen to me, a person whom she just met!

This intervention did not make this experience easy for Amy nor did it make her stop crying in that moment. However, it did make it bearable for her, and it provided her with a foundation for coping that she and her family needed for future procedures and treatments. Importantly, it also modeled for her parents that the anxiety they brought into the room fueled Amy's anxiety so much that she tuned them out completely to adhere herself to me, who was calm, quiet, and nurturing. Amy did progressively better as her treatments went on. It took a couple of months for her to rebuild a trusting relationship with her parents and for me to teach her parents how to facilitate coping techniques for her before she was able to do a spinal tap without having to be held down. But I am proud to say that we did eventually get there.

Most parents lack significant knowledge of hospital events to accurately and adequately prepare their children for a doctor's visit or admission to the hospital. Sometimes a phone call to the doctor's office is necessary for parents to gather information about their child's upcoming visit. A parent needs to gather information regarding the sensory aspects of the visit: What will my child see, feel, hear, smell, and so on? Having this information will decrease the child's level of anxiety and fear of the unknown in an unfamiliar medical setting.

Patients of all ages, who are cognitively capable of understanding a simple explanation, need an accurate, reassuring, and developmentally appropriate explanation of the illness, hospitalization, surgery, procedures, and treatment plans. Children are especially vulnerable to fear if they do not have a clear understanding of their surroundings. They often dramatize and weave fantasies to try to make sense of their situation and of the information they have been given.

Parents need to be prepared for what they are going to see because their anxiety and fear can generate anxiety and fear in their child. Children can pick up on a parent's non-verbal cues of fear and concern very easily. They know you and all of your expressions. If they sense that you are afraid, upset, or concerned and you do not explain your demeanor to them in a simple way, their anxiety will increase as they feel that "something must be really bad for Mommy to be so upset." They could worry that you are withholding information or not sharing the whole truth about the medical situation. So, if parents acquire a simple, elementary understanding about the procedure or treatment, they are more likely to feel comfortable and capable of assisting their child through the procedure and providing him with a model for effective coping.

Five Key Elements of Effective Preparation and Education

1. Effective preparation and education includes five key elements. The first element of effective preparation is learning the developmentally appropriate language. Use simple and soft speech and "Straight Talk," which I will describe in this chapter.

2. The second element is facilitation of emotional expression so that a child has the opportunity to reveal prior knowledge of medical events, misconceptions, fears, and/or anger.

3. The third element is giving and explaining information age-appropriately. Without age-appropriate explanations of the procedural and sensory information, the child cannot learn to cope with experiencing the event.

4. The fourth element of effective preparation is emotional support given from someone on the health care team whom the child has gotten to know and trust (like the individual who prepared her for the procedure). Facilitating a child's emotional expression requires an understanding of the child's state of mind.

5. The fifth key element of effective preparation is providing a safe environment for the child to ask questions. By safe environment I do not necessarily mean a physical space, but more of a child friendly place and a safe relationship with the parent or the person preparing her. For example, an appropriate place to prepare a child

for surgery is in a quiet play environment, like at a table when the child is coloring or playing quietly. It would not be appropriate to discuss and prepare your child while he is waiting for his turn at a batting cage. This environment is too distracting, and you will be unable to capture his attention. A child needs to feel safe that he will not be demeaned or laughed at for asking a silly question and to not worry that he will get in trouble or be mocked for expressing his fears or concerns. The bottom line is that he needs to feel supported during this process, without fear of being embarrassed, belittled, or having his concerns dismissed as unimportant or unrealistic.

Preparation for a procedure should be done within a timeframe that allows the child to process the new information and express feelings of concern both verbally and non-verbally through play with a parent. Parents are partners in the preparation process, assisting their child so there is true understanding of the events of the procedure or treatment. By participating in the preparation of their children, parents are not only supporting their child but also really thinking about the medical information the doctor gave them so that they can interpret it and devise a non-threatening way to explain it to their child. This process is invaluable for the parent because it forces a full understanding of the procedure and reduces his or her own fear and anxiety.

Choosing Appropriate Language

The words that are chosen to explain something to a child will have a tremendous impact on how the child will react to the explanation. Many words have multiple meanings, which can be very confusing to a little one without mastery of the language. Choosing words is tricky because what words and phrases are helpful for one child may be threatening for another. For example, consider if you were to tell a child, "The doctor is going to take a stool collection." The child might think, *"Why would he want to collect little chairs, and how am I going to get him one of those?"* A clearer explanation is to use a term that the child is familiar with, such as "poop" or "BM." So, a much better explanation would be, "The doctor needs you to go poop into this cup. He will test the poop, which can tell him what is going wrong with your body. Once he knows what is wrong, he will be able to help fix it."

The following section lists some examples of confusing explanations for medical procedures and common medical terminology that have a tendency to confuse and frighten children. In addition, I have given suggestions for ways to address these topics in a clearer and less threatening way. I call this "Straight Talk."

Anesthesia

Confusing explanation for anesthesia:

The doctor is going to put you to sleep.

A child may think:

You mean like my dog was put to sleep. That means that I will never come back.

Straight Talk explanation:

The doctor is going to give you some medicine called anesthesia. I call it sleepy medicine because it makes your body sleep so you won't feel anything. The sleepy medicine will also make your mind sleep so you won't remember anything either.

Dressing or Bandage Change

Confusing explanation for a dressing change:

The doctor is going to come and do a dressing change.

A child's understanding:

Why are they going to undress me? You mean I have to be naked?

Straight Talk explanation:

The doctor is going to come and change your bandages, to give you new or clean ones.

Contrast or Dye

Confusing explanation for contrast or dye:

The doctor is going to inject dye into your veins.

A child might wonder:

Am I going to die?

Straight Talk explanation:

The doctor is going to put a medicine called "contrast" into the small tube in your hand. This is going to help her see your body more clearly in the picture that will be taken of the inside of your body.

Urine

Confusing explanation for urine:

I need to collect your urine.

A child may think:

You're in? In what? Where?

Straight Talk explanation:

Use more familiar terms like pee-pee, saying: I need you to go pee-pee in this cup so the doctor can test it to see what is going on inside your body.

Injections or Shots

Confusing explanation for shot:

The doctor needs to give you a shot.

A child's understanding:

With a gun? Why are you mad at me? When people get shot, they get really hurt. Are they trying to hurt me?

Straight Talk explanation:

The doctor is going to give you some medicine with a poke; it is a small needle that gives your body the medicine it needs, and it is the only way to give you this type of medicine. They cannot give it to you any other way.

CAT or CT Scans

Confusing explanation for CAT scan: We are going to give you a CAT scan.

A child's interpretation:

> *You mean a kitty cat? You are going to put a cat on me? Is it going to scratch me?*

Straight Talk explanation:

> The doctor is going to take a very clear picture of the inside of your body with a CT scan machine. It is a big camera, which looks like a big donut. You will get to go through the center of the circle so they can take a picture of you from all sides.

PICU (Pediatric Intensive Care Unit)

Confusing explanation for PICU:

> You are going to go to the PICU (pronounced, "PICK YOU").

A child wonders:

Pick you? Why did (or didn't) they pick me? What did I do wrong?

Straight Talk explanation:

You are going to the Pediatric Intensive Care Unit. That means that you will probably have your own nurse who will be with you a lot and will be right there if you need her to make sure you are safe and aren't hurting. They call it the PICU. But they are not picking anyone or any part of you.

PACU (Post Anesthesia Care Unit)

Confusing name for the place where you go to recover after undergoing anesthesia:

You are going to the PACU (pronounced "PACK YOU").

Straight Talk explanation:

They are taking you to the Post Anesthesia Care Unit where the nurses observe you while your sleepy medicine wears off. They call it the "PACU." But they are not going to pack you or pack anything.

ICU (Intensive Care Unit)

Confusing explanation for ICU:

We are going to visit the ICU.

A child hears:

I see you? I see you too.

Straight Talk explanation:

Same as above. Explain in simple terms what the letters ICU stand for— Intensive Care Unit.

Operating Room (OR) or Treatment Room Table

Confusing explanation for OR, exam (or treatment room) table:

Please get up on the OR table.

A child is concerned:

I am not allowed to get up on tables at home. Am I going to get in trouble if I get up on a table?

Straight Talk explanation:

The doctor needs you to get up on this narrow bed; they sometimes call it a table, but it is more like a bed.

Stretcher or Gurney

Confusing explanation for stretcher:

Get up on this stretcher.

A child hears:

Stretch her? Isn't that going to hurt?

Straight Talk explanation:

You need to get up on this bed. Look, it has wheels like a car so they can move it around.

O_2 or Gas Mask

Confusing explanation for gas or gas mask:

> The doctor is going to give you anesthesia in a gas mask.

A child wonders:

> *You mean someone is going to pour gas into the mask? I won't be able to breathe. What? I didn't pass gas!*

Straight Talk explanation:

> You are going to get some sleepy medicine that is a different kind of air that you will breathe. It may smell like _____ [ask doctor]. It will make you feel very sleepy. Once you are asleep, then the doctor can start the procedure or surgery.

Radiology Procedures

Confusing explanation for taking a picture or X-ray CT and MRI:

> The doctor needs to take a picture of you.

A child wonders:

Where is the little camera; should I smile? Can I see the picture?

Straight Talk explanation:

Say, The doctor is going to take a picture of the inside of your body with a very special camera. Then, describe the camera to the child, what it looks like, and what kind of sounds and movements it makes.

IV Starts

Confusing explanation for IV:

The nurse is going to place an IV.

A child hears:

Ivy? The plant?

Straight Talk explanation:

The nurse needs to give you an IV. This is a small tube that is put into your vein [make sure you explain vein] because that is the fastest way to give you medicine that will make you feel better. The nurse will have to give you a poke in your arm. The needle guides the tube is right where it needs to go. When the tube is in place, the needle is taken out. All you will see is a soft tube and some tape on your hand.

IV Care

Confusing explanation for IV care:

The nurse is going to flush your IV.

A child wonders:

Flush it down the toilet?

Straight Talk explanation:

The nurse needs to clean out your IV tubes. She does that by adding a saline, which looks like water. They call that flushing the IV, which is flushing the medicines through the tubes to clean them.

Moving Rooms

Confusing explanation for being moved to another patient room:

You are going to be moved to the floor.

A child wonders:

Why do they want to put me on the ground?

Straight Talk explanation:

They are going to move you to another room [give brief explanation]. They call that unit "Peds," which is short for Pediatrics. We also call this "The Unit" or "The Floor."

Poor Vein Access

Confusing explanation for the nurse not being able to access a vein:

He or she is a difficult stick, or he or she has bad veins.

A child thinks:

She called me bad and difficult. I am not bad. Am I? Maybe it's my fault they keep poking me.

Straight Talk explanation:

Your veins are small, and the nurse is having a difficult time finding them. You have little veins that are difficult for the nurse to see.

As you can see through these examples, the way something is explained to a child can greatly affect his thoughts and perceptions of the given situation. We need also be aware that communicating to children in soft, non-threatening words is necessary for the child to be able to cope with the information without the child perceiving the situation as terribly threatening.

In the medical setting, there are a number of threatening words that medical professionals use in their daily language that are confusing or seem scary to the majority of adults, especially those for whom English is their second language. For example, more times than not, I have heard nurses refer to needle insertion as a "stick" or a "prick," both threatening and harsh words in my mind. When I think of the word "prick," I think of running into a rose bush. *Ouch!!!!* With this in mind, it makes perfect sense that I wouldn't want to have this done to me! The same goes for the word "stick." This has a negative meaning for me because I sew, and many times I have stuck my finger with a needle. We all know this hurts! So let us remember that words to describe medical events can have negative and threatening overtones, which can scare a child whether he understands the meaning of the word or not. Therefore, I advocate for softening your speech in describing the medical environment to children. This again means describing the procedure to a child in a clear, non-threatening arena where he feels safe to ask questions and express concerns without worry or guilt. The following chart lists some additional examples of words and phrases spoken loosely in the medical environment that can be threatening. Also included are corresponding words or phrases to replace them with to ensure maximum understanding and coping. Your speech should be simple and soft; I creatively call this, "Simple, Soft Speech."

[1] Threatening or Negative Words	Clearer or More Positive Replacement
Cut, slice, incision	Make a small opening
Burn	Will feel warm or hot
Stick or prick	Poke (or "pokie" for the little kids)
As big as _____	Smaller than _____
Discharge	Go home
Taste or smell bad	Will taste or smell different or unusual
Blown vein	Vein isn't working right now
Say goodbye to your parents	Say "see you later" to your parents
As long as _____	In less time than it will take to _____
Ambulate	Walk
Hurt or pain	Sore, achy, or tight
Respirate	Breathe
Restrain or hold you down	Help you hold your body still if you cannot do it by yourself
Injection or shot	Needle poke
Catheter	Special tube
Isolation	You have to stay in your room
Inpatient	Patient in the hospital
Outpatient	Patient visiting the doctor in a clinic or office
Put you to sleep	Give you sleepy medicine, or medicine that will help your body sleep
Take vitals	Measure your temperature and measure your blood pressure

[1] Adapted from John Wolfer, Joy Goldberger, Richard Thompson, Lisa Redbum, Lesley Laidley, and Laura Gaynard, *Considerations in Choosing Language: Psychosocial Care of Children and Hospitals*, Clinical Practice Manual from the ACCH Child Life Research Project (Rockville, MD: Child Life Council, 1998).

Helpful Sample Preparations

The remainder of this chapter describes a variety of sample ways that I have prepared children for various procedures. It is important to note that each of these sample preparations is a guideline for you. The intention is not to provide a script that you would simply read to your child. Rather, you must adapt the information to the child's level of understanding and the differences in the procedure itself. The amount of information that I provide is not appropriate for every child. Older children need more information than younger children and also need a more precise explanation. In addition, every medical center is different and every doctor has his or her own techniques, so make sure you have precise information about the step-by-step process. Only in this way are you able to accurately describe it to your child. It is so important for you to gather information from the doctor *prior* to preparing your child for any medical event. Remember, these are just some examples to give you an idea of what a medical preparation is like.

Sample Preparation #1: Surgery

- ✓ *You are going to have an operation. It is also called a surgery.*

- ✓ *When you get to the hospital, you will go to an admitting/waiting area where mom and dad have to fill out papers to sign you in.*

- ✓ *Then we will go to another room; usually this is a big room where you will get to see some other patients who are also having an operation. This is the room where patients go to get ready for the Operating Room (OR). Here you will meet your nurse.*

- ✓ *The nurses are really nice. They help make you comfortable as you get ready to go to the OR. Your nurse will give you a bag for your clothes and give you a special gown to wear.*

✓ *We will bring your special toy [tell her which one] to play with while we are waiting for the nurses and doctors.*

✓ *Remember, the doctor told us that you would have to get a poke (injection) before you go to the OR. The nurse will have to put in a small tube called an IV catheter. An IV is a tiny tube that is placed into one of your veins that allows the doctors to give you special medicine during your surgery. It is very important that you hold your arm still for the nurse. She has to aim her needle for your vein, and if she misses, sometimes she has to do it over again. Don't worry, it doesn't take long. It feels like a pinch, but I will be there with you the whole time.*

✓ *Then the nurse will give you a mask for you to breathe in. It gives you oxygen to help your breathing. It may smell funny, but it doesn't hurt at all.*

✓ *A nice person who wears clothes like a doctor will come and get you when the doctors are ready for you in the OR. Your mom and/or dad can walk with you, but they cannot go all the way into the OR.*

✓ *In the pre-op area and in the operating room, the doctors and nurses wear special clothes, hats, and masks that are super, super clean to keep the germs away from you.*

✓ *A special doctor called an anesthesiologist is going to give you some special medicine that will make you feel very sleepy. It will make your body and your mind fall asleep so that you don't feel any hurt or owies during your surgery. This medicine is called anesthesia, but that is hard to remember so I call it "sleepy medicine."*

✓ *The sleepy medicine will make you forget your surgery. When you wake up, you won't remember anything about your surgery. Some kids ask, "Mom, when are they going to start my surgery?" after it is already over.*

✓ *When your surgery is done, the doctor or nurse will wake you up in a room called a Post Anesthesia Care Unit. For short, many hospitals call it the PACU. Your mom and dad may come in to this room and see you as soon as your surgery is over. Your throat might feel dry and scratchy. But that will go away soon.*

✓ *You still will be really sleepy and won't remember anything about your surgery because you will be asleep the whole time! If you feel sore after your surgery, the nurse gives you special medicine that helps take the pain away.*

You will have to wait here in the PACU for a while. The nurse will slowly give you ice chips and then maybe a drink. It depends on how you are feeling. Sometimes the sleepy medicine makes your tummy sick, so they give you food and drinks really slowly so you don't ever feel the need to throw up.

Sample Preparation #2: IV Insertion

✓ *You need to have a special medicine.*

✓ *The kind of medicine that you need is not a pill or syrup that you can drink.*

✓ *The doctor is going to use something called an IV (not "ivy" the plant). IV stands for "in the vein." The doctor needs to give you medicine into your vein [show child where his veins are]. That is where this special medicine needs to go to help you feel better.*

✓ *To give you IV medicine, you will get a poke into your vein. It will feel like a pinch for just a short time. But I know that the nurse is going to need your help. You need to help the nurse by staying still. When you are still, he or she can see your veins and get the medicine there pretty quick. It will only take less than a minute if you can help by holding completely still. We can work together to think and talk about your favorite place, or we can look at a book to make the time go by faster.*

✓ *Most kids say that the poke feels like when a brother, sister, or friend pinches you. That is all. Can you close your eyes and imagine someone pinching you? That is what it will feel like.*

✓ *Most kids say that it is much less scary if they can close their eyes, or look away toward their mom or dad, and think of something fun, like pretending to blow out birthday candles or blow bubbles.*

✓ *When the nurse is finished, you will have a little tiny tube in your vein that will be taped down so you won't bump it or knock it out. That tiny little tube allows the medicine to get right where it needs to go, and you will start to feel better.*

Sample Preparation #3: Bone Marrow Aspiration

✓ *You are going to have a test that is called a bone marrow aspiration. The reason you have to have this test is because the doctors need to find out what is causing you to feel sick [or for an older child, give appropriate reason].*

✓ *During this test, the doctor is going to give you a poke [say two pokes if an anesthetic is given] in your lower back, above your bottom (or butt).*

✓ *Before the procedure starts, the nurse will put some cream on your back where the doctor is going to do the poke. The cream is going to help take the feeling away on your skin. It is called numbing. The doctor wants to numb your skin so that you will not feel as much ouchie when they have to do the poke.*

✓ *Most kids say that they do feel the poke a little. But they say that it doesn't feel like a pinch like an IV poke does; they say that it feels like something heavy is pushing on their back, like a person sitting on them. But remember, the cream the nurse puts on your back is going to help you not feel it so much.*

✓ *A lot of times the doctors give you even more medicine so that you won't feel the poke during this test. [Make sure you know what kind of sedation the child will be getting and what the effects of that sedation are. Will it make him forget? Will he be asleep? Will he still feel some pain? Then be honest about how the sedation will help him. Don't tell the child he is going to be asleep if he is not.] The doctor will give you this extra medicine called oral versed [or name whatever sedation your doctor chooses to use] with either a poke or into your IV. This medicine's job is to numb your skin, make you sleep, make you forget, make you relax, and so on.*

✓ *It sometimes sounds silly to have to get a poke so that you won't feel the poke for the test, but most kids say that they really like that medicine because it works like magic to take that next ouch away.*

✓ *The doctor is going to ask you to lie on your belly or over a pillow so that he can see where he needs to give the poke.*

✓ *The test itself doesn't take very long. What takes the longest is for the doctors and nurses to set up. They want to make sure that your bed is really clean and that anyone touching you is really clean.*

✓ *First the doctor is going to spend time getting all set up.*

✓ *He has to get dressed before he starts the test. He wears a gown to cover his clothes and a hat to cover his hair. He also wears special clean gloves.*

✓ *He also is going to clean your back. He does this six times! First he cleans three times with an orange soap, then three times with a clear soap. This is to make sure your skin is totally clean.*

✓ *Then he will give you the first poke to give you the extra numbing medicine to help you with the second poke. This will take less than a minute. Then he will do the second poke for the test. This poke also only takes a minute or so.*

✓ *Finally, he will collect the fluid that he needs to get from your back into a tiny little tube. Once he gets what he needs, you are done! The nurse will put a small bandage on your back; it's called a "pressure dressing."*

Sample Preparation #4: Blood or Lab Draws

✓ *The doctor needs to do some tests on your blood to make sure that your body is healthy or to determine what medicines to give you to make you feel better.*

✓ *We are going to a place called the lab.*

✓ *In the lab, there are people who are experts at getting blood from our bodies. They are called phlebotomists. Don't worry; they won't take too much, just the right amount for the doctor to be able to run some tests on it.*

✓ *First you can sit on my lap, and the phlebotomist will tie a big rubber band around your arm, giving it a tight hug. She also will tell you to make a fist, like you are going to punch. This helps her see your veins better. Veins are these blue things that carry the blood around our bodies [show yours].*

✓ *The phlebotomist will look for a vein that looks good to take some blood from. Don't worry; your body will not miss the blood that is taken.*

✓ *Then, she will clean your arm with an alcohol pad. This feels cold.*

- ✓ *Finally, she will give you a poke on your arm. The poke is usually right in a vein on the arm, opposite the elbow.*

- ✓ *The poke goes by really fast. It feels like a pinch. She will get the blood needed and then take out the needle.*

- ✓ *During the poke, it is best if you look away from your arm and look at me, into my eyes. I will tell you a story and hold you to help you relax.*

- ✓ *[Parents: It is very important to remember that during this time you lock eyes with the child and speak in a calm, quiet, soothing tone, no matter how loud the child or the environment is. Your child will come down to your level and listen to you.]*

- ✓ *Remember, I will be there the whole time. It is OK to cry if you are scared, but the most important thing is that you hold your arm still. You don't want to move and have an accident with the needle if the poke is put in the wrong place. Can you hold still by yourself, or do you think you may need a* nurse or Mommy to help you hold your arm still?

✓ The entire procedure will only take a minute or two, and the poke will take seconds! Once the nurses get the blood they need, then we can leave the lab and go home.

Sample Procedure #5: Ideas for Supporting Children When Taking Oral Medicines

Say to the child: "I have to give you some medicine soon. When would you like to take it—before lunch or after lunch?"

By stating that you must give the child medicine, it lets her know that she has no choice in the matter and that there isn't any behavior that is going to change the situation. Allowing her to choose when she can take the medicine, however, gives her some choice and helps her feel some independence in making decisions and participating in her own care. Many parents make the mistake of asking the child, "Do you want to take your medicine now?" Most children are likely to say no. Then what do you do? At that point, *you'll have to move to exerting authority and control over the child, which makes her upset and feel powerless. This often leads to a parent/child fight or leads to crying and/or resistance on the child's part. This situation can easily be avoided by approaching a child that needs to take her medicine with respect and empathy.*

If a child is refusing to take the medicine, ask her why and show that you care by trying to help her. Many times children have valid reasons for not wanting to take the medicine. I have come across many reasons for not wanting to take medicines, for example, "It tastes yucky. It doesn't help anyway. It makes me throw up. It hurts my mouth. It makes me feel sleepy." Once you understand what is behind the resistance, you can help by asking the doctor to change the medicine (if possible) or asking the pharmacist if the medicine could be given another way that could make the child feel more comfortable. Oftentimes medicine can be given as a pill, syrup, or an IV med. Ask.

In the hospital, I once worked with a nine-year-old boy who was refusing to take his pain medicine. He was visibly in a lot of pain. He looked miserable and was in tears. He was alone in his room; his father had to go to work. The nurse was insisting that the child take the pain medicines and told him it would make the pain stop. The child got more upset and was in tears. His nurse paged me to come and talk to the child and to try to get him to take his medicine. After I introduced myself and expressed that I was there to try to help him, he told me that his nurse was forcing him to take medicine. He was very upset at her. After I listened to him and validated his feelings, we were able to sort this out. Within a short time I was able to establish a relationship with this boy in which he felt safe enough to reveal the reason for his refusal to take his medicine. He didn't want to take the medicine because it made him sleepy. But he didn't want to fall asleep because his mom was scheduled for a visit and he wanted to spend time with her. Through his tears, he told me that he didn't see his mom too often because his parents were divorced and didn't get along. He lived with his father, who restricted visits with his mom.

My heart sank for this poor little guy. Not only was he sick and in pain, he was alone and felt like he had no one to help him. Immediately, I spoke with the physician and requested that the pain medicine be changed to something that did not cause drowsiness. The physician agreed to change the order. The pain subsided, and the boy was able to stay up and visit with his mom.

Once I knew that his mom would be visiting that day and that the visit was important to him, I was able to provide them with activities and games that the two of them could play together to make for a more special visit.

Chapter 6 Review

1. *Children need to be prepared for their medical procedures, both invasive and non-invasive.*

2. *Address topics in a clear and less threatening way. I call this "Straight Talk."*

3. *Tell children step-by-step what is going to happen to them to alleviate fear of the unknown and to avoid misconceptions.*

4. *When talking to children about medicine or medical events, use simple and soft speech.*

5. *Effective preparation and education includes five key elements: learning developmentally appropriate language, facilitating emotional expression, explaining information, giving emotional support, and providing a safe environment for the child to ask questions.*

Therapeutic Play

Carrie

"Play for young children is not recreation activity. It is not leisure-time activity nor escape activity. Rather, play is thinking time for young children. It is language time, problem-solving time. It is memory time, planning time, investigating time. It is organization-of-ideas time, when the young child uses his mind and body, his social skills, and all his powers in response to the stimuli he has met."

—James L. Hymes, Jr.,
Child development specialist and author

Run. Jump. Crawl. Throw. Clap. Sing. Bang. Roll. Climb. Pretend. Imagine. Draw. Bump. Build. Create. Sort. Zoom. Push. Pull. Hop. Bounce. Bonk. Feel. Wiggle and jiggle. These activities are a child's primary modes of coping. Playing! Play can act as a learning tool for children to help them familiarize themselves with and cope with the medical environment. Unstructured or "free" play can be informative, fun, and relaxing to a child. It allows children to resolve problems and helps them formulate positive attitudes toward adults and the medical environment, which could later facilitate adjustment to future medical experiences, dental visits, and hospitalizations. In addition, play allows children to express themselves without the use of verbal language, to which a child is limited. The famous Greek philosopher Plato once said, "You can discover more about a person in an hour of play than in a year of conversation." Play can reveal the true feelings and emotions of an individual, while facilitating learning and coping with feelings and emotions.

The idea of providing "therapeutic play" means that a person would provide children with pleasant and psychologically beneficial experiences. This is typically the role of a Play Therapist in a therapy setting or a Child Life Specialist in a hospital setting. If your medical center has a Child Life Specialist, it is beneficial to utilize these professionals to ensure that your child is receiving age-appropriate education about his situation. A Child Life Specialist will introduce coping skills and teach your child to use these coping techniques in all life situations. If a Child Life Specialist is not available to you, you as a parent or caregiver can perform this function—with the knowledge and understanding you learn from this book about the importance of play and how you can provide these opportunities for your children.

Play is essential for children to cope with and make sense of the environment. In play, children are able to cope with fear, difficult emotions, and situations of heightened anxiety that are so common in the medical environment. Play is where children can escape from reality and take on another role if they wish. Playing the role of a doctor, for example, allows a child to assume the role of authority and gain a sense of power. While role-playing, children can also revisit past medical situations that may have been difficult for them. This gives them a second chance to handle things differently if they choose and also allows them to practice coping. Play is a place where children can utilize skills and independence and try to make sense of information and situations in an environment that is familiar and safe. In play they are capable, in control, and effortlessly functioning in a developmentally appropriate place. In other words, they are acting like a kid!

Children can also use play to familiarize themselves with the medical environment by playing with medical equipment. By this, I mean touching it, poking it, banging it on the floor, exploring it with their mouth, or doing whatever they do to test out a new object. This is called *exploration* or *familiarization*. Many children I have met are terrified of medical instruments, even items as non-threatening as a strip of paper measuring tape. The child is completely out of his element. He is being approached by an unfamiliar person (the nurse) in an unfamiliar environment (the hospital), with an unfamiliar object (the measuring tape). It is easier to understand your child by removing yourself from the immediate situation. In this case, while watching your child throw a tantrum over a 24-inch paper measuring tape, think about what it would be like to be touched with an object you have never seen before. You don't know what it is, how it is going to be used, whether it will hurt or not, and you are unsure of the strange person who is approaching you with it. I know for me, given the opportunity to check it out on my own terms, my own timeline, in an environment that is comfortable for me, and then given the chance to ask questions, I would have a much easier time. The one and only way to provide this for children is to provide an opportunity for them to play with these foreign objects. Allow time for them to play with these items on their terms, and definitely be available to answer their questions.

Now you can take familiarization one step further and allow the child to make a special doll or teddy bear become a shadow buddy. A shadow buddy, in a child's imagination, becomes a patient just like her that will mimic whatever your child is going through or having done to her. Remember my cereal bowl story from the first chapter? Well, after I fell on that brick, I remember bleeding everywhere and holding my arm in a towel on the way to the doctor. I remember being terribly afraid. I thought my arm was coming off. My mom had to take me to a doctor that I did not know. I was so panicked that the doctor threatened to have my mom leave the room if I wouldn't calm down and let him look at my arm. I immediately stopped my outburst, I didn't move, and I let him do his job, out of fear that he would take away my mom and hurt me when she was out of the room. Now, I am sure that if you asked that doctor or his nurses, this tactic worked in making me hold still for him to examine my arm. What they will never know, however, is how that insensitive threat affected me and changed the way I viewed medicine and doctors. I suffered a traumatic experience and vividly remember the fear I felt. To this day, 30 years later, I still remember his name and the way he looked in his short-sleeved blue doctor's smock and brown tortoise-shell framed glasses. I remember him as the mean doctor who threatened me. Sadly, I probably will remember him this way for the rest of my life.

My mom didn't really know what to do either (but if you ever run into her, never tell her that I said that). She had every intention of helping me through this experience and was sensitive to my fear, but she didn't know how to calm me down and didn't really know or understand why I was so afraid. If I had been old enough or wasn't so anxious, I could have told someone that the objects on the tray terrified me. Someone possibly could have taken the time to explain what was going on. Then, if I had been given the time to see and touch the doctor's equipment and been able to ask questions about what was on his tray, I think things would have gone much better.

After I had gotten the stitches in my arm and my mom took me home, she got some needle and thread and stitched up my most treasured possession, my Cabbage Patch Kid named Lana Liza. She placed stitches in the doll's arm and bandaged her up, just like my bandage. She let me play with the bandages and participate in taking care of Lana. As a result, I carried the doll around *everywhere* while I had my stitches! I felt understood by my mom; I felt loved and felt I was not alone. When it came time to go back to the doctor's office to have the stitches removed, my mom took off Lana's bandages, showing me what the doctor was going to do to take the stitches out. By playing with me, she prepared me for the experience of how the doctor was going to remove my stitches. She let me remove Lana's bandages, snip off some of Lana's stitches, and play with her and her bandages until I was done.

That follow-up visit, I don't remember quite as much. However, I do remember trusting my mom and what she told me about what the doctor was going to do. I also remember that I was excited to get my bandages off, just like Lana Liza did. I know that I sat still. I allowed the doctor to take the stitches out and did not require an army of nurses to hold me down. *Preparation matters; understanding and validating a child's fear matters.* I know this truth firsthand.

I also know firsthand the validity and importance of play as a means to teach; play also allows children to express feelings and thoughts that they are unable or unwilling to verbalize. My experiences as a child affected me so profoundly, I made it my life's work to do everything I can to help children through scary times at the doctor and to show parents that their role in their child's medical experiences is much bigger than they think it is.

Let your child play! Use this method to help your children cope with any anxiety-evoking situation that presents itself in their lives. It is important to give them some individual time to play and explore, but sometimes, join in with them and be a playmate. The safe environment and the mastery that a child feels while playing paves an open road for communication and heart-to-heart talks with you. In this setting, a child is more likely to ask questions and truly display her feelings and anxieties. These moments with a child are truly precious and can enlighten you to a side of your child that she has never been able to communicate to you in any other way.

Chapter 7 Review

1. *Play is a child's primary mode of coping. Play can act as a learning tool. It can be informative, fun, and relaxing. In addition, play allows children to express themselves without the use of verbal language, to which children are limited.*

2. *Play is essential for children to cope with and make sense of their environment.*

3. *Play can be used as a modality to familiarize children with the medical environment. By playing with medical equipment, children are learning about it, making these items less scary.*

The Use of Positive Reinforcement and Rewards

Zachery

It seems that in our nation today, there is much talk about the use and overuse of "rewards" as a means to control our children or to get them to behave. I agree with the use of rewards as a means to obtain expected behaviors in children—if and when this technique is used correctly. Sometimes it is appropriate to offer praise and rewards; we will talk about the appropriate way to provide this without allowing your child to act inappropriately and end up controlling you.

If a child earns the reward (keyword here being "**earns**"), it is OK to give a small reward from time to time. However, overuse of this idea creates a feeling of entitlement within children, where they will expect a reward every time they behave. The rewards for good behavior, ideally, should be the child gaining the intrinsic rewards of building self-esteem, gaining control of his emotions, learning to cope with difficult situations, and/or being able to control fearful or anxious emotions. These rewards can be gained through support, praise, and encouragement.

A system for rewards needs to be set up in advance. For example, if the child is going for a painful or invasive procedure, criteria can be set for him to meet so as to earn a small treat after the procedure is over. Here is an example of the criteria that could be set for the child: "You need to keep your body still and keep your hands and feet to yourself. In addition, you need to be respectful to the doctor and nurses. If you don't think you can stay still by yourself, you can ask a parent or a nurse to help you hold still. It is OK to be scared and to cry. You can ask for support and help to accomplish these tasks, and I will help you."

These are reasonable criteria to ensure the child's safety and the safety of the nurses or doctors performing the procedure. These are tangible behaviors that you are telling your child you want to see, and if you do see these behaviors, he will earn a reward. To give the child the option of asking for help is so empowering for him, because children who have their eye on the prize want to earn it, but may need help holding their bodies still or may need help with distraction so that they are able to earn their prize and feel successful.

If the child is screaming, hitting, kicking, not cooperating with the doctor or nurse, or using inappropriate language, the reward should not be given! It seems like a simple concept, but it is more difficult than it seems. Many times we as parents are too general, like when we say, "I will give you a lollipop if you behave." This is too general. What exactly does "behave" mean, and who determines what is considered good behavior? Good behavior to a parent can mean something entirely different to a child. For a child, getting through a procedure without hitting someone is considered "behaving." For a parent, we often expect more. So clarifying exactly what behavior you expect to see is helpful to keep you and your child on the same page.

Determining expected behaviors in advance is also essential. Parents commonly will make their behavior judgment or their decision whether to give a reward based on their own feelings of guilt and their desire to rescue a child after watching him go through something scary or possibly painful. It is difficult not to want to rush in and provide something that will make him happy after watching him cry or experience pain. No parent wants to see his or her child crying or terrified. This empathy we feel toward our children sometimes gets in the way of being able to make an appropriate judgment, so we give them a reward whether we see the behavior we expect or not. *Wrong!* This is so confusing to children. They don't understand that you are empathetic toward them or their situation and that is the reason why they received the reward. Rather, they hear you saying, "If you behave, you can have a toy." They get the toy, then they evaluate: "Hmmm. I screamed at my mom, hit her, and told the doctor that I hated him. These must all be acceptable behaviors; after all, I got a lollipop for doing these things."

So what can you do to practice the proper use of this rewards technique? When you are preparing your child for the procedure or event, you can tell him that he is going to get a poke and that you know getting a poke is scary and difficult for him. You then tell him what kinds of behaviors are acceptable. For example, you can say, "If you are scared, it is OK to squeeze my hand" or, "If you are scared or hurt, it is OK for you to cry." Then you can tell the child that you will be there for him to hold his hand or offer hugs. Finally, it is then you can bring up that there will be a reward for him if he earns it. It is vital to clearly tell him what he must do to earn his reward.

It is important to establish reasonable expectations. Reasonable expectations are expectations that are logical for your child's developmental age and ability to cope with difficult situations. For example, it is not reasonable to expect a two-year-old to hold still for a shot without help; neither should a fearful teen be expected to either. For these children, a reasonable expectation is, you must sit down and let the nurse help you hold still. In addition, they can say that they are mad or that they don't like it, but they cannot say hurtful things to other people.

The reason why this concept is so important for you to understand is because many doctor's offices provide positive reinforcement to the children as a way of saying, "I am sorry I had to poke you." Doctors or nurses will give the children praise when it is deserved, but I also have heard many say, "Good job" or "You were so brave" when the child was screaming and kicking or when the child's behavior was awful. Therefore, we cannot rely on the doctor or nurse to teach our children how to behave appropriately at the doctor's office. They will likely get a toy or a sticker from the doctor's "prize box" just for going to the doctor. Many of these items are given upon completion of the visit, regardless of the child's behavior. That is why you must prepare yourself so you don't wind up giving your child mixed messages, which can lead to more inappropriate behaviors.

Be honest with your child. If a reward is going to be given no matter how a child behaves, you might as well say, "I am going to give you a reward when you are done. It doesn't matter how you act; you get it for just completing your doctor's appointment. You don't have to behave." This may sound absurd, but at least it is consistent and you are not sending the child a mixed message.

Offering appropriate praise to a child in similar situations is used incorrectly even more frequently than incentives. For example, let's look at a child who is getting a shot. Remember, I have witnessed this many times and have seen children do all sorts of ill-willed, nasty things to their parents and their doctors and nurses. I have seen children kick, scream, hit, bite, push the doctor away, or curse at their parents and/or the doctors and nurses, yet at the completion of the procedure, the parent will say, "You did such a good job" or offer some sort of praise. On one hand, this is perfectly understandable. We sit there, watching our children go through something that is terrifying or pain-evoking, and we have no idea what to say to comfort them. Yet on the other hand, we end up giving unearned praises because we feel bad for them, lacking the understanding of how confusing this is. Again, by praising inappropriate or violent behavior, it sends the child the message that this type of reaction and behavior is acceptable *when it is not.* If hitting, kicking, biting, and screaming or cussing at people are not acceptable behavior in the home or on the playground, then these are not acceptable just because the child is afraid. Being consistent will further support children's understanding of appropriate behaviors in daily life situations.

Let me share an example of this consistency and use of rewards. My son was going to the doctor to get a flu vaccine. He thought that he was going to get the nasal mist. Unfortunately, the doctor told him that because of his asthma, he was unable to get the vaccine nasally and would have to get a shot. Meanwhile, his little sister was going to get the nasal mist. When the nurse left the room, I did my best to talk to him and remind him about the procedure of getting a shot. I talked about what it was going to feel like and how long it would take, but he wasn't listening. He was just saying over and over that he didn't want it. He was taken by surprise, totally off guard, and he was not happy. He began to cry and was unable to listen to me as I tried to help him calm down. He was upset; he was resistant and needed to be partially restrained.

When the nurse came in, Zachery was flailing his arms around and was not cooperative. I was shocked because he usually does really well. I got my first experience of feeling embarrassed that he was being so uncooperative and throwing a tantrum. I just held him and reassured him as best I could. I apologized to him about the surprise the doctor gave us that time and told him that I wished he could have received the nasal vaccine. I told him that I loved him, that even though I was disappointed in the way he acted, I understood that he was scared. Driving home, we spent the majority of the 30-minute drive talking about what we could do when we are scared, other than hit and be uncooperative with the nurse.

I usually give my kids a small surprise when they do cope well with getting a shot. I get them a milkshake, a lollipop, or a small toy. My kids really thrive on earning treats, and I only offer them for one thing—shots. And so, it wasn't surprising that Zachery expected a toy because he got a shot. Poor little guy was so sad when I told him that he did not earn a treat and would not be getting one. I wanted to give him one so badly just to make him smile, but I didn't. I wanted to show him that he had to earn a reward and explained to him repeatedly just how to do that.

One month later, we had to go for the second dose. I was not looking forward to this at all. I spoke to him the morning of the shot; we went over the step-by-step procedure of what the nurse was going to do. We talked about the feeling of a shot and about the shot he had received a month prior. I reminded him of what I expected of him to earn a toy this time. I gave him two tangible behaviors that I expected. I told him that it was OK to be scared and it was OK to cry. But I also expected him to cooperate with the nurse, to do what she told him, and to keep his arms and legs still.

I am happy to say that he did great with the second shot. He was like a different kid! He was nervous, but he was confident that he could get through it and earn the toy. He allowed me to hold him, and he listened attentively as I talked to him and told him, step-by-step, what the nurse was doing. When the nurse started counting down to the injection, he began to squeeze my hand. He was so brave. He didn't move, he didn't cry, and he smiled after, so proud of himself. We drove to Target immediately afterward, and I gave him $5 to pick out a toy. He deserved it.

The proper use of rewards is essential so that you can avoid creating a child who behaves solely for a reward or the promise of a reward. If you are going to use a reward, you must set an attainable goal to be achieved. Goals that would be considered attainable are, for example, if the child is able to hold still for the doctor or if he lets the nurses help him hold his body still without fighting. On the other hand, an unattainable goal would be to expect a fearful child to go through a medical visit without crying by saying he can have a reward if he doesn't cry.

Once the goal is set, if the child achieves it, he obtains the reward. If he doesn't meet the goal, the reward cannot be given. You will have one disappointed child on your hands, and you should expect to have to deal with tears and possible tantrums. This should be expected; it is how children handle the disappointment of not pleasing their parents and not getting a sought-after reward. Don't give in. Tell the child that he did not get the reward this time, but that he can try again next time. Then quickly try to redirect the child toward something else, like, "Let's go home and play with your special toy" or "Why don't we listen to your favorite song when we get in the car?"

Chapter 8 Review

1. *The use of rewards is appropriate in the medical setting from time to time, if this technique is used correctly.*

2. *Rewards should not be given if they are not truly earned.*

3. *Determining expected behaviors in advance is essential so the child will know right away if he or she has earned a reward.*

Conclusion

There are eight basic principles that can help you facilitate a more positive experience for children in the medical setting:

1. Relationship building

2. Facilitating coping

3. Becoming a tower of trust

4. Listening and providing empathy

5. Introducing the medical procedures

6. Providing non-threatening information in an age appropriate way

7. Valuing Play

8. Rewarding desired behaviors

By reading this book, you have already taken the first step to helping your child build an age-appropriate understanding of the health care environment. Actual scenarios have been presented to help you learn how to provide support to your child during stressful and anxiety-evoking situations, which will help him cope throughout his entire life. In this way, you are taking part in building a community of emotionally healthy children, who then will become emotionally healthy adults able to cope during times of stress and armed with the tools necessary to provide empathy and comfort to their own children.

By providing your children with age-appropriate introductions to the doctor and medical environment, you are introducing something strange and foreign in a safe and non-threatening way. This ultimately will enable more positive experiences with the medical environment. Providing this information in a caring, empathetic way will also show your child that you care about her feelings, understand her concerns, and acknowledge her fears as normal. When a child has an understanding parent, whom she can count on to answer any question openly, honestly, and on her terms, she then identifies the parent as the person to go to for help and support. What parent wouldn't want that kind of relationship with their child?

Having the tools to cope with heightened anxiety and fear is essential to a child developing a healthy way of handling difficult situations effectively. Some children needlessly fail to develop coping capabilities to the fullest because of an illness, handicap, emotional imbalance, or other conditions. My hope is that, after reading this book, you now have the skills to safeguard your child's medical experiences to help him develop effective coping strategies. Once you have identified your child's coping style, you can make a huge difference in helping a scared child through a difficult time.

Acting as a strong tower of trust, or creating and maintaining a trusting relationship with your child, is an essential component of parenting during times of fear, frustration, and loss of control. A child cannot calm his mind and body enough to listen to you, and really hear you, if he does not trust that what you are saying is going to have validity. If he does not have confidence in you as someone able to provide the physical and emotional support he needs, he will feel lost, alone, and helpless. These are the feelings that lead to those tantrums, screaming fits, and uncontrollable behaviors that embarrass parents. Acknowledge the child's feelings; let him know that you understand and still love and accept him. Keep in mind that a child loses trust easily. Most parents assume that their child trusts them; however, that is not always the case. Ask yourself these questions: "When my child is upset or crying, does he turn to me for comfort or help?" and "Do my attempts to calm her and ease her fears help?" If the answer is no, then creating this bond is possible—and easier than it seems. Remember these five steps: Admit, Address, Reassure, Check in, and Remind. Following this simple formula will develop a newfound trust and allow children to feel the comfort and ease that come with knowing someone is on their team and looking out for them.

When a child feels that his voice is being heard and understood, he is comforted. This can foster an environment for positive coping, learning, and further development of trusting relationships. Sometimes children do not have the verbal skills or the strength to communicate their needs to you. Sometimes they are not even sure what they want. They just know that they are not comfortable with their current situation and need help making sense of it. Listening to their questions and searching for the hidden meaning can help you address the concerns that the child is unable to verbalize. Advocating for your children's needs and voicing their concerns when they cannot do so themselves can provide relief for them in knowing that someone understands them enough to take their feelings into account when making decisions on their behalf.

Children require developmentally appropriate education and communication about medical events to avoid misconceptions and misunderstandings formed while trying to make sense of the foreign words they hear and unfamiliar objects they see in the medical setting. Consider using the list of basic developmental needs in Chapter 5 when preparing your child for a visit to the doctor. Identify these needs and help your child understand what to focus on when trying to communicate. In addition, communication tips are provided in Chapter 5 to assist you in speaking to your child in a safe and non-threatening way.

Step-by-step preparation about new experiences is key to providing positive learning experiences that help a child feel confident in new situations. The five key elements to effective preparation are using developmentally appropriate language, facilitating emotional expression, explaining information, giving emotional support, and providing a safe environment for the child to ask questions. This is difficult to do if you lack the information to adequately prepare your child. You must have this information to be accurate, so *don't be intimidated* to call the doctor and ask specific questions that will address sensory aspects of the visit (that is, what the child will see, feel, hear, smell, taste, and so forth).

I cannot reiterate enough how important play is to the emotional health of a child. It provides the perfect environment for preparing a child for a medical event. It is not merely a recreation activity. It is everything to children. This is where they learn new skills, cope with emotions, experiment with new objects and ideas, and express themselves. They need play opportunities all the time, especially when they are sick or going through a difficult time. This is the reason so many hospitals offer children playrooms, not to prevent them from being bored, but to provide them a place to escape from the realities of their situation and be kids. A playroom or a play environment is safe and non-threatening to a child. It gives the child a sense of control and mastery over his environment, which can help a child build on his self-esteem. In introducing anything new to a child, allow her to touch it, manipulate it, push, pull, twist, and hit it. When a child familiarizes herself with the new objects, it makes the objects less scary and foreign. Medical instruments are no exception.

Children are well endowed with the qualities and potential to promote their development. As a parent, our job is to help them develop, to understand them, and most important, to enjoy them. Children's growth and development are predictable. They are strong and will adapt to a loving and trusting environment.

With this book, I hope that I have prepared you and given you the appropriate information that you need to make a difference in your child's life. I know that these simple principles can help your children learn to deal with new, stressful, and possibly frightening situations that they will encounter not only in the medical environment, but also as they grow and move through the experiences of life. I wish you and your children a healthy life and stress-free medical experiences. I hope that by reading this book, you feel more confident and prepared to make that reality happen. I also wish you luck and success in nurturing your relationship with your child to a place where they will still be looking to you for support when they are 35. I love you, Mom.

For this end, I have given you the tools and provided insight into your child's thoughts about the health care environment. I think that some would say I have written myself out of a job. But rather, I believe that I have enlightened millions of parents about the field of Child Life and how its professionals think, care, and nurture children in the health care system.

My life's work has been helping and supporting children during times of fear and/or heightened anxiety, mostly in the medical setting. Now that I have had these 10 years of experience in this setting, my eyes have been opened to the vast opportunities to further my mission and find other ways to help children globally. Giving parents the tools to help their children through difficult situations and procedures is an integral part of my plan to better equip our children in dealing with difficult life situations and helping parents establish trusting relationships with their children that will last a lifetime.

It gives me purpose and pleasure to be able to help and support a scared child and watch his demeanor transform before my eyes when I can provide the developmentally appropriate information and coping tools he needs to get through the fear and feel successful in overcoming challenges.

Through this book, I am hoping to reach more children across the world. I am committed to donating half of the proceeds to ZOE International, a Christian non-profit organization that is dedicated to combating trafficking of children globally, especially in the sex trade. ZOE is dedicated to rescuing children sold or who are at risk of being sold to prostitution, in slavery, orphaned, or at risk of becoming victims of other heinous crimes. ZOE Children's Homes serve children 0–18 years of age. ZOE's homes nurture a child's spirit, soul, and body in a strong Christian atmosphere where they provide the highest quality academics and receive excellent health care and nutrition. They also provide continuing education for the children over 18 years of age. At ZOE, children are loved unconditionally and taught the Word of God by highly trained staff.[2] My mission is to help support them.

"Fighting for Those Who Cannot Fight for Themselves"

Psalm 10:18, Psalm 82:3–4

---

[2] Taken from www.gozoe.org